Essentials in Ophthalmology

Series Editor
Arun D. Singh

More information about this series at http://www.springer.com/series/5332

Mark S. Humayun
Editor
Lisa C. Olmos de Koo
Associate Editor

Retinal Prosthesis

A Clinical Guide to Successful
Implementation

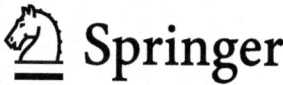 Springer

Editor
Mark S. Humayun, MD, PhD
Roski Eye Institute
Institute for Biomedical Therapeutics
University of Southern California
Los Angeles, CA
USA

Associate Editor
Lisa C. Olmos de Koo, MD, MBA
University of Washington Eye Institute
Seattle, WA
USA

ISSN 1612-3212   ISSN 2196-890X   (electronic)
Essentials in Ophthalmology
ISBN 978-3-319-67258-8   ISBN 978-3-319-67260-1   (eBook)
https://doi.org/10.1007/978-3-319-67260-1

Library of Congress Control Number: 2017964093

Printed on acid-free paper

This Springer imprint is published by Springer Nature
The registered company is Springer International Publishing AG
The registered company address is: Gewerbestrasse 11, 6330 Cham, Switzerland

Preface

The Argus II retinal prosthesis is the first device of its kind to both earn a CE mark for use in Europe and to be approved by the United States Food and Drug Administration (FDA) as a humanitarian use device (HUD). Since that time, it has been successfully implanted in hundreds of patients suffering from profound blindness, uniquely transforming and enriching their lives. With the introduction of the Argus II, what was once considered the realm of science fiction has at last become reality.

As an approved medical product entering the commercial marketplace, there has been intense interest focused on the optimal implementation of this device in the fields of ophthalmology and visual rehabilitation. Much discussion has been generated as to how it should best be used to help those afflicted by retinitis pigmentosa and related conditions. This book is intended as a useful and practical guide, primarily oriented toward ophthalmic practitioners involved in retinal prosthesis implantation and postoperative visual rehabilitation. However, it may also be of great interest to affected patients and their loved ones who have a scientific background or inclination.

We have selected the top experts in the field as chapter authors, many of whom have been working on the Argus project for decades. We are fortunate that much of the groundwork for the development of the Argus retinal prosthesis was done here at our home institution, the USC Roski Eye Institute and at the USC Institute for Biomedical Therapeutics, where the first experimental implants were performed nearly 15 years ago. Since that time, USC has partnered with Second Sight Medical Products as well as top ophthalmic centers across the country and the globe to conduct device clinical trials and, ultimately, to make the Argus II available to the public.

The organization of this book is straightforward. We begin with a brief history of retinal prostheses as well as some background on bioengineering considerations. We then delve into the most practical aspects of device implementation: patient selection, surgical technique, and expected outcomes, both clinical and functional.

Finally, we focus on future directions for this exciting device. The book concludes by a chapter on other methods in development to restore sight. It is our hope that this guide will help eye care professionals around the world in their mission to restore sight to those blinded by retinal degeneration, those who need it most.

Los Angeles, CA   Mark S. Humayun, MD, PhD
Seattle, WA   Lisa C. Olmos de Koo, MD, MBA

Contents

Contributors

Antoine Chaffiol, PhD Institut de la Vision, Sorbonne Universités, UPMC Univ Paris, Paris, France

Yao-Chuan Chang, PhD Department of Biomedical Engineering, University of Southern California, Los Angeles, CA, USA

Laura Cinelli, MD Department of Surgery and Translational Medicine, Eye Clinic, University of Florence, Florence, Italy

Gislin Dagnelie, PhD Department of Ophthalmology, Johns Hopkins University School of Medicine, Johns Hopkins Hospital, Baltimore, MD, USA

Jens Duebel, PhD Institut de la Vision, Sorbonne Universités, UPMC Univ Paris, Paris, France

Gregory Gauvain, PhD Institut de la Vision, Sorbonne Universités, Paris, France

Devon H. Ghodasra, MD Ophthalmology and Visual Sciences, University of Michigan, Kellogg Eye Center, Ann Arbor, MI, USA

Olivier Goureau, PhD Institut de la Vision, Sorbonne Universités, UPMC Univ Paris, Paris, France

Ninel Gregori, MD Bascom Palmer Eye Institute, Department of Ophthalmology, University of Miami Miller School of Medicine, Miami, FL, USA

Allen C. Ho, MD Clinical Retina Research Unit, Wills Eye Hospital, Retina Service, Philadelphia, PA, USA

Mark S. Humayun, MD, PhD Roski Eye Institute, Institute for Biomedical Therapeutics, University of Southern California, Los Angeles, CA, USA

Christelle Monville, PhD Université Evry Val Essonne, Paris, France

Lisa C. Olmos de Koo, MD, MBA University of Washington Eye Institute, Seattle, WA, USA

Serge Picaud, PhD Institut de la Vision, Sorbonne Universités, UPMC Univ Paris, Paris, France

Stanislao Rizzo, MD Department of Surgery and Translational Medicine, Eye Clinic, University of Florence, Florence, Italy

José-Alain Sahel, MD Institut de la Vision, Sorbonne Universités, UPMC Univ Paris, Paris, France

Centre Hospitalier National d'Ophtalmologie des Quinze-Vingts, DHU Sight Restore, Paris, France

Fondation Ophtalmologique Adolphe de Rothschild, Paris, France

Department of Ophthalmology, The University of Pittsburgh School of Medicine, Pittsburgh, PA, USA

K. Thiran Jayasundera, MD Ophthalmology and Visual Sciences, University of Michigan, Kellogg Eye Center, Ann Arbor, MI, USA

James D. Weiland, PhD Department of Biomedical Engineering, University of Southern California, Los Angeles, CA, USA

USC Roski Eye Institute, Institute for Biomedical Therapeutics, University of Southern California, Los Angeles, CA, USA

Lan Yue, PhD USC Roski Eye Institute, Institute for Biomedical Therapeutics, University of Southern California, Los Angeles, CA, USA

David N. Zacks, MD, PhD Ophthalmology and Visual Sciences, University of Michigan, Kellogg Eye Center, Ann Arbor, MI, USA

Chapter 1
Retinal Prostheses: A Brief History

Lan Yue, James D. Weiland, and Mark S. Humayun

An Overview of the Proof-of-Concept Studies and Visual Prostheses

The eighteenth century witnessed the early explorations in the physiological responses to electrical stimulation, accompanying unraveling of the mystery of electricity. In 1775, LeRoy created light sensations in the blind by passing electrical currents around the head. In 1780, Galvani discovered twitching in the muscles of dead frogs' legs that were struck by electricity. Two decades later, Volta reported receiving a jolt in the head and then hearing bubbling sound when he inserted two electrodes in his own ears. Over the past two centuries, these early experiments at the electrode-tissue interface have progressively evolved into a variety of programmable, chronically stable bio-electronic implants, such as visual prosthesis, cochlear implant, pacemaker, deep brain stimulator, and bladder control, that serve to regulate or restore certain physiological functions (Weiland and Humayun 2008; Niparko 2009; Beck et al. 2010; Kringelbach et al. 2007; Van Balken et al. 2004). These devices are built upon the similar basic principles of the extracellular stimulation of the nervous system, though

L. Yue, Ph.D.
USC Roski Eye Institute, Institute for Biomedical Therapeutics, University of Southern California, Los Angeles, CA 90033, USA
e-mail: lyue@usc.edu

J.D. Weiland, Ph.D.
Department of Biomedical Engineering, University of Southern California, Los Angeles, CA 90089, USA

USC Roski Eye Institute, Institute for Biomedical Therapeutics, University of Southern California, Los Angeles, CA 90033, USA
e-mail: jweiland@med.usc.edu

M.S. Humayun, M.D., Ph.D. (✉)
Roski Eye Institute, Institute for Biomedical Therapeutics, University of Southern California, Los Angeles, CA 90033, USA
e-mail: humayun@med.usc.edu

© Springer International Publishing AG 2018
M.S. Humayun, L.C. Olmos de Koo (eds.), *Retinal Prosthesis*, Essentials in Ophthalmology, https://doi.org/10.1007/978-3-319-67260-1_1

they target different neural circuits. Among them, a bioelectronic visual prosthesis is a device that is intended to restore functional vision in the visually impaired patients by electrically stimulating the neurons of the visual signal pathway.

Early visual prosthesis experiments investigating the susceptibility of the visual cortex to electrical stimulation were separately reported by Foerster in 1929 (1929) and by Krause and Schum 2 years later (1931). They discovered that direct application of the electrical pulses to the visual cortex elicited perception of light spots termed "phosphenes" in both sighted and blind subjects. More specifically, their pioneering work showed that (1) point stimulation of the cortex produced localized light perception, (2) location of the phosphene in the visual field roughly corresponded with the site of stimulation, and (3) visual cortex remained functionally capable of generating light sensation after deprivation of visual inputs for years.

These findings laid the groundwork for the cortical visual prosthesis, the first prototype of which was developed and implanted by Brindley and Lewin (1968) in the late 1960s. The prosthesis contains 80 intracranial platinum electrodes encapsulated in a silicone cap, each connected to an extracranial radio frequency receiver that is pulsed wirelessly by an oscillator through induction. A 52-year-old woman blinded from glaucoma and retinal detachment received the surgical implantation of the device and reported to see phosphenes when the electrodes were activated. The brightness of the phosphenes was dependent on the pulse frequency and duration. Location of the phosphenes in the visual field was correlated with the location of the stimulating electrode, and phosphenes were spatially distinguishable when the electrodes 2–4 mm apart were simultaneously activated. As the first clinically tested visual prosthesis prototype, the Brindley and Lewin device further demonstrated the possibility of using a chronic implant to restore sight and perhaps more importantly, its architecture has the continued influence on the various visual prosthetic systems that would appear decades later. In the 1970s, Dobelle et al. (1974) carried out a modified design that incorporated a television camera to feed the stimulating electronics with the visual input. This device enabled a blind subject to see discrete phosphenes and to recognize simple patterns including large letters.

Aside from the visual cortex, electrical stimulation at the other locations along the visual pathway also produces perception of light. In 1969, Potts and Inoue (1969) recorded electrically evoked potentials in retinitis pigmentosa patients and in normally sighted volunteers, when stimulated with cornea electrodes. In more recent years, electrical prostheses interfacing with the visual system, respectively, at the level of retina, optic nerve, and geniculate nucleus have been described (Dowling 2009; Veraart et al. 1998; Pezaris and Eskandar 2009). There is no consensus on the ideal site of stimulation as the option is largely governed by the pathophysiology—each type of prosthesis is limited to treat blindness arising from the damages upstream but not downstream of the stimulation site. For example, retinal prostheses would serve best for the outer retinal degeneration, e.g., retinitis pigmentosa (RP) and age-related macular degeneration (AMD), where the inner retina and the rest of the visual pathway remain relatively intact and functional, but it is not indicated for diseases such as glaucoma in which the optic nerve is completely damaged or blindness due to damages to the higher visual centers in the brain.

Retinal prosthesis has recently garnered the most attention among the different visual prosthesis types perhaps for the following reasons: (1) in comparison with the optic nerve in the back of the eye and visual centers in the brain, the retina is easier to access for surgeries and is associated with lower surgical risks; (2) retinotopic mapping is well preserved in photoreceptor-degenerated retina, and therefore stimulation site in the retina is highly correlated with the location in the visual field, enabling less complex conversion of the spatial information from the visual scene to the physiologically interpretable stimulation pattern; and (3) originating electrical signaling in the retina takes advantage of the computational power of the remaining visual circuitry, therefore will be likely to better mimic the normal visual processing. This chapter will focus on the historical aspects of the representative retinal prostheses, briefly accounting the background, the advancement, and the future directions.

Retinal Degenerative Diseases and Treatment Options

Retina is a light-sensitive stratified neuronal tissue that lines the back of the eye. It is ~0.5 mm in thickness, and the retinal neural network consists of several layers of cell bodies and their neural processes of dendrites and axons, as illustrated in Fig. 1.1a. The retinal pigment epithelium (RPE) cell layer, lying adjacent to the neural retina, is involved in recycling the visual pigments and maintaining the health

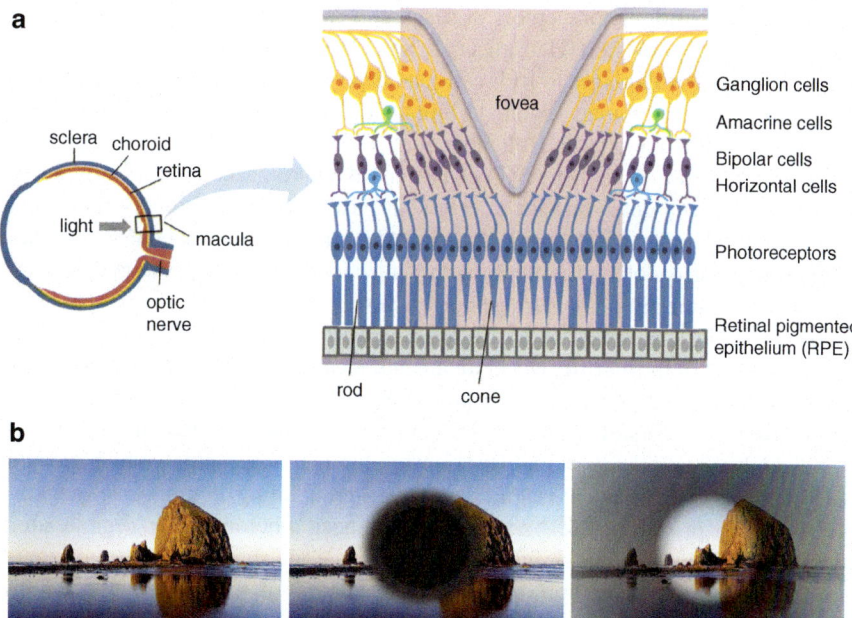

Fig. 1.1 Retina and retinal degenerative diseases. (**a**) Schematic representation of the stratified structure of neural retina. *Pink-shaded area* represents the macular region. (**b**) Effects of retinal degeneration on visual field. *Left*: Visual field of a normally sighted subject; *Middle*: Central vision loss in macular degeneration. *Right*: Peripheral vision loss in retinitis pigmentosa

of photoreceptors, the light sensor in healthy retina. Visual signals, initiated at the photoreceptors, sequentially travel through the bipolar cells and ganglion cells and propagate to the higher visual centers in the brain via the optic nerves (axons of the ganglion cells). Signals also receive lateral modulation from horizontal cells and amacrine cells, as part of the neural processing in inner retina. As shown in Fig. 1.1a, cell distribution profiles are very different in central vs. peripheral retina. Cone photoreceptors are densely packed in the macula and especially the fovea, while rod photoreceptors predominate in the peripheral region.

Retinal degeneration involving progressive deterioration and loss of function of photoreceptors is a major cause of permanent vision loss (Busskamp et al. 2010; Curcio et al. 2000). AMD and RP are the two most prevalent forms of retinal degenerative diseases. Epidemiologic studies show that the onset of AMD occurs predominantly in the elderly, while RP has an earlier onset in children and young adults (Wong et al. 2011).

Together, they account for millions of cases of blindness and visual impairment worldwide. Figure 1.1b shows representative patterns of vision loss in AMD and RP. AMD begins by primarily affecting photoreceptors in macula, leading to blurred central vision. As AMD progresses, the blurred area typically grows larger, and the patient develops blind spots (scotomas) in the center of the visual field (Jackson et al. 2002). AMD affects 30–50 million people globally and more than two million in the United States alone (Bressler 2004; Friedman et al. 2004).

Most common form of RP (rod-cone degeneration) starts with progressive degeneration of rod photoreceptors in peripheral retina resulting in loss of peripheral vision and night vision (Hartong et al. 2006; Wells et al. 1993). Degeneration of rods is followed by damages to RPE cells and deterioration of cones, resulting in the visual decline from "tunnel vision" to blindness. RP is estimated to affect 1.5 million people in the world (Den Hollander et al. 1999).

There is no cure for either AMD or RP, and the current therapies mostly aim to slow down the cell death and the concomitant vision loss. Nutritional supplements have been used to prevent the progression of AMD and RP (Richer et al. 2004); anti-VEGF (vascular endothelial growth factor) injections and lasers have been used to slow neovascularization or destroy abnormal vessels in wet AMD (Heier et al. 2012; Wood et al. 2000). However these treatments are very limited in blocking or reversing the progression of the disease. Novel treatments such as new drugs, gene therapy, and cell transplantation are under investigation (Beltran et al. 2012; Rakoczy et al. 2015).

In advanced stages of photoreceptor degeneration, inner retinal circuitry is also significantly altered. Lack of regular input from the photoreceptors, which are nonresponsive or absent, leads to significant neural remodeling. A number of negative physiological processes are heralded by advanced photoreceptor degeneration, including neuronal and glial migration, extensive neurite sprouting of the horizontal and amacrine cells, formation of the synaptic microneuromas, and evolution of a fibrotic glial seal that increasingly isolates the remaining retina from RPE and choroid (Fariss et al. 2000; Marc et al. 2003). Despite reorganization and cell loss, the inner retinal neurons largely retain the capacity for signal transmission. Morphometric analyses have shown that, based on the nuclei count, nearly 90% of the ganglion cells survive wet AMD and the ganglion cell density in dry AMD does not differ significantly from that in normal eyes, even in retinal areas with virtually no remaining photoreceptors (Kim et al. 2002; Medeiros and Curcio 2001). Morphologic studies in severe human RP patients reveal moderate preservation of inner retinal neurons: 70–80% of the bipolar cells and 25–40% of the ganglion cells (Santos et al. 1997; Humayun et al. 1999; Weiland et al. 2011). Inner retinal preservation suggests the possibility of vision restoration by establishing a stimulation mechanism that bypasses the damaged photoreceptor layer and directly interfaces with the remaining inner retinal neurons.

Fundamentals of Electrical Retinal Stimulation

In bioelectronic retinal implants, an electrode array is placed in close proximity to the retina, forming an electrochemical interface with the physiological saline. Current, injected by the stimulating electrodes, passes through the retinal tissues to the return electrode, either locally placed on the array or at a distant location. Current delivered into the extracellular region causes charge redistribution on the cell membrane of the retinal neurons. In cathodic stimulation, negative charges build up on the outside of the membrane underneath the electrode, driving the intracellular movement of the positive charges from the neighboring compartments to this region, resulting in strong membrane depolarization close to the electrode and weak hyperpolarization further away. Firing of action potentials is initiated when membrane depolarization exceeds a threshold.

For electrical stimulation of a complex neural network such as retina, charge redistribution on the membrane of axons, soma, and dendrites will all contribute to the depolarization of the retinal neurons. The axon initial segment (AIS) of the RGC is located at the proximal end to the soma and contains a high density of sodium channels. Extracellular stimulation localized to different compartments of the retinal ganglion cells shows that the AIS has the lowest activation threshold, followed by other axonal sections and the soma, with the dendrites exhibiting the highest threshold to the electrical stimuli (Tsai et al. 2012). At the subcellular level, action potentials initiated at one neuronal element may propagate to another, significantly affecting the temporal and spatial response dynamics of the cell. For example, it has been demonstrated that activation of the passing ganglion cell axons that is in close proximity to the electrode may result in the perturbation of the membrane potential that travels orthodromically toward the distal end of the axon and antidromically toward the soma (Tsai et al. 2012). The antidromically propagated depolarization may evoke spiking of the soma that is located further away from the electrode, causing diffused activation map of the retina. At the network level, synaptic transmission in inner retina shapes up the indirect activation of the ganglion cells and presumably in the modulation of the ganglion cell signaling.

Stimulation waveform is identified as a key factor in the response pattern of the retina. Variations in the pulse strength, duration, and frequency have exhibited influence on the population selectivity, activation spatial profile, and stimulation efficiency (Tsai et al. 2012; Weitz et al. 2014, 2015; Nanduri et al. 2012). The choice of stimulation waveform also needs to factor in the electrochemical safety considerations. It has been found in the stimulation of the monkey cerebral cortex that a monophasic current pulse, consisting only of a cathodic or an anodic phase that is not charge balanced, creates damages, including loss of electrical excitability and tissue viability, whereas no damage was noted with biphasic charge-balanced stimulation of similar strength (Lilly et al. 1952, 1955). It is revealed by these and other studies (Brummer and Turner 1975) that a symmetry of electrochemical processes serves to maintain the integrity of the electrodes and to avoid net charge accumulation at the electrode-tissue interface which will eventually lead to unsafe chemical reactions. Retinal implants today mostly employ charge-balanced biphasic waveforms consisting of a cathodic phase for stimulation and a charge-balancing anodic phase for accelerated electrode discharge.

Development of the Retinal Prostheses

Significant progress in the field of the retinal prostheses was made at the turn of the twenty-first century. In the late 1990s, Humayun et al. (1999) demonstrated, in acute settings, that electrical current delivered from a multi-electrode array to retina generated phosphenes in blind subjects. The subjects were able to report the location of the perception in their visual field, and track perception as the electrode was moved to different locations in the retina. In another proof-of-concept trial of acute retinal stimulation, RP patients reported the ability to discriminate two separate stimulation points (Rizzo et al. 2003). These important pilot studies revealed retinotopic correlation between the stimulation and the phosphenes generated, demonstrating the feasibility of using a multi-electrode array to elicit visual percepts that, to some degree, reflect the stimulation pattern. Since then, the field of retinal prosthesis has rapidly evolved, spawning the Argus II implant (Second Sight Medical Products, Inc.) and the Alpha-IMS implant (Retina Implant AG) that are commercially available, as well as several other prototypes that are currently in clinical trials.

A retinal prosthesis functions as an integral system that consists of multiple components. Typically, it contains an image acquisition device, an image processor, a stimulator chip, and an electrode array. Images acquired from the visual field are directly or indirectly translated into the current stimuli that are delivered by the multi-electrode array to the retina. In a camera-electrode system, images are captured by a video camera and converted by a specialized processor to the stimulation patterns that are subsequently delivered to the implanted stimulator chip. In contrast, in a photodiode system, the visual information, sometimes preprocessed, is directly detected by the electrode-coupled photodiodes to generate electrical stimuli. When needed, the power and data transmission between the external part of the device and the implant often take the form of radio frequency (RF) telemetry and/or optical link that is minimally invasive. Despite similarities in the basic architectures

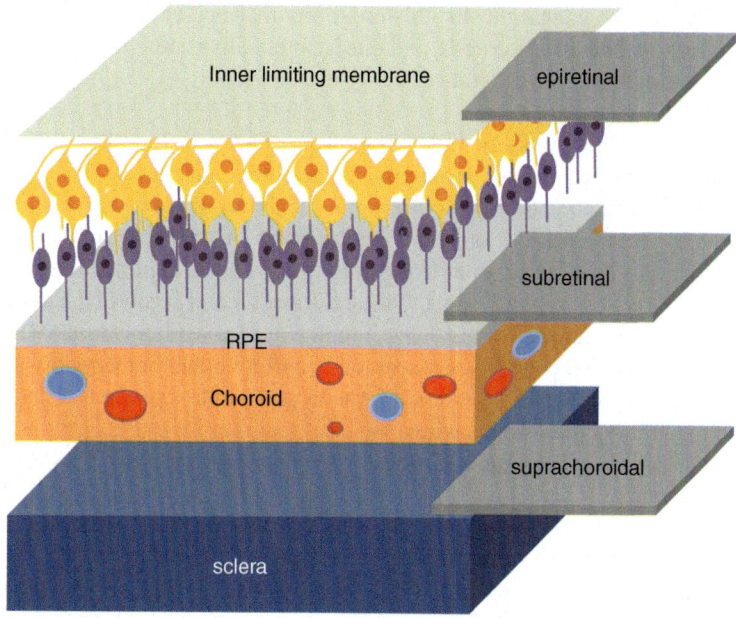

Fig. 1.2 Illustration of the implantation sites of the epiretinal, subretinal, and suprachoroidal prostheses. Ganglion cells (*yellow*) and bipolar cells (*purple*) are shown, and damaged/eliminated photoreceptors are not shown

of different retinal prosthesis systems, their specific designs diversify, largely depending on the locations where the electrode array is implanted and the complexity of the implanted electronics. Three main types of retinal implants have been developed: epiretinal prostheses, anchored to the inner surface of retina; subretinal prostheses, embedded between the retina and RPE/choroid; and suprachoroidal prostheses, implanted between the choroid and sclera (Fig. 1.2).

Epiretinal Prostheses

Epiretinal prostheses, sitting on the innermost layer of retina, have several advantages:

1. Ease of surgery: the prosthesis contacts the retina on the inner surface that is accessible from the vitreous, and the vitreous cavity makes room for surgical maneuvers, reducing risks of mechanical damage to the retina.
2. Heat dissipation: besides choroidal perfusion, fluid in the vitreous cavity serves as an additional heat sink that enhances the removal of the heat generated by the electronics of the implant, lowering thermal risks for chronic use (Opie et al. 2012).

3. Proximity to the ganglion cells: this proximity makes it easier for the device to directly stimulate ganglion cells, and this is potentially useful in extended retinal degeneration where inner retina circuitry is altered.

The potential drawbacks of the epiretinal prostheses include the difficulty of implanting the array in close proximity to the retina and the perfused/distorted visual percepts due to undesired activation of the axons of passage, which may be overcome by lengthening the stimulation pulse width. A large share of the efforts in retinal prosthesis development has been directed toward the epiretinal type. Groups that have reported farthest progress in this arena are Second Sight Medical Products (SSMP) Inc. in Sylmar, California, USA, Intelligent Medical Implants (IMI) GmbH (acquired by Pixium Vision SA, France), and EpiRet GmbH in Germany. Devices from these three groups all use external cameras and wireless power and data transmission to avoid transcutaneous wires.

Two generations of devices, Argus I and Argus II, were developed by SSMP. Argus I is a first-generation epiretinal prosthesis approved for an investigational clinical trial by the United States Food and Drug Administration (FDA). Studies on the Argus I demonstrated the safety of long-term stimulation, motivating the development of the more advanced Argus II retinal implant, which received European Union approval (CE Mark) in 2011 and FDA market approval in 2013. Argus I was a modified cochlear implant and strictly an experimental device, while Argus II was designed as a retinal prosthesis intended for commercial use.

The basic operations of the Argus series systems are similar, both consisting of a miniature camera mounted on a pair of glasses, an external video processing unit (VPU) worn by the user, as well as an extraocular and an intraocular implant that are interconnected via a transscleral cable. The camera captures visual scenes and sends the information to the VPU for advanced pixelation and processing (Fig. 1.3a). The hermetically packed extraocular electronics, along with a transceiver antenna, converts the RF signals it receives wirelessly from the VPU to the electrical pulses whose amplitude corresponds to the brightness of the local pixel (Fig. 1.3b). Stimulation pulses are delivered by the cable to the intraocular electrode array that is attached to the retina via a tack. On the user side, the most prominent difference between the two devices perhaps lies in the number of electrodes. The array of Argus I and Argus II contains 16 and 60 electrodes, respectively. The Argus I electrodes are 250 and 500 μm in diameter, whereas the Argus II electrodes have a reduced diameter of 200 μm (Fig. 1.3c). Compared with Argus I, the Argus II array not only contains a higher electrode (pixel) density for increased spatial resolution but also covers a larger retinal area to accommodate a greater visual angle—an estimated increase from $10° \times 10°$ for Argus I to $11° \times 19°$ for Argus II.

Between 2002 and 2004, Argus I was implanted monocularly in six subjects blinded by RP (De Balthasar et al. 2008; Mahadevappa et al. 2005; Horsager et al. 2009). Between 2007 and 2009, a total of 30 subjects (29 with RP and 1 with choroideremia) received the Argus II implant in the United States and Europe (Ho et al. 2015). Details of the outcome of these clinical trials will be presented in Chap. 5. Overall, safety was observed with both devices, and all subjects perceived light

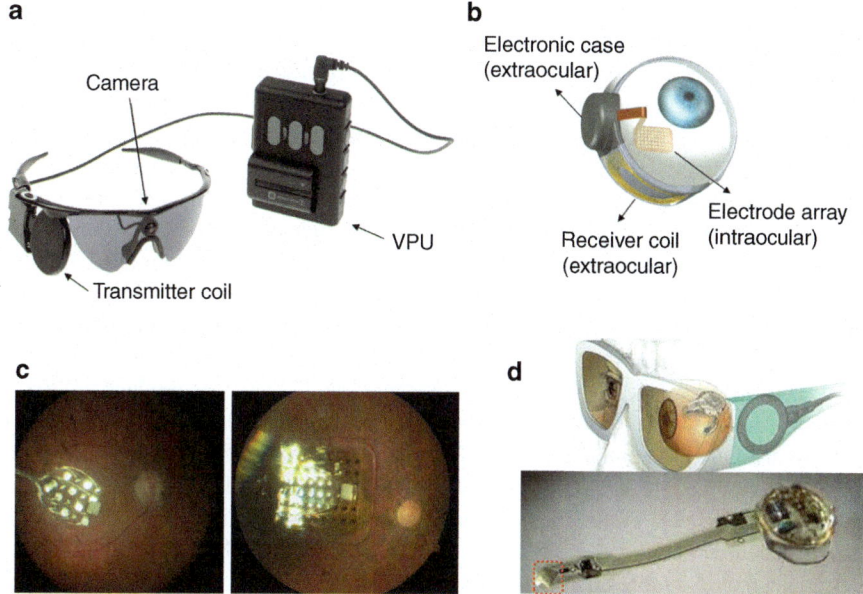

Fig. 1.3 Epiretinal prostheses. (**a**, **b**) External (**a**) and implant (**b**) part of the Argus II system. (**c**) Electrode array of the Argus I (*left*) and Argus II (*right*) implant, containing 16 and 60 electrodes, respectively. (**d**) Schematic drawing of the IMI system and the implant prototype. The stimulating array is circled in *red* (images reprinted from Hornig et al. 2007)

when the device was activated and they could perform visual spatial and motion tasks after a short period of training. Furthermore, the restored visual acuity, to a large extent, depends on the spatial resolution of stimulation—the best grating visual acuity restored by Argus I and Argus II is 20/3244 and 20/1262, respectively. As the first retinal implant with regulatory approval, Argus series systems offer exciting opportunities to study prosthetic vision in a relatively large cohort of patients. Results from clinical trials provide strong evidence that electronic retinal implant is effective in restoring meaningful vision to patients blinded by photoreceptor degeneration.

The IMI retinal implant consists of a visual interface, a pocket processor and a retina stimulator (Hornig et al. 2007). IMI operates similar to Argus II and the difference lies in the wireless transmission. Distinct from Argus II that uses a single pair of RF transceiver coil for power and data transmission, IMI employs two wireless links: RF transmission for power and infrared (IR) optical link for data. The IR transmitter, consisting of IR LEDs, is embedded in the visual interface and located in front of the eye. The IR receiver lies intraocular, as part of the implant. The optical link allows for high data rate, and it can be actively interrupted by simply closing the eyelid, as an instinctive response in normally sighted people. The prototype IMI carries 49 iridium oxide electrodes that are connected via a cable to the retina stimulator electronics encapsulated by polyimide (Fig. 1.3d), without additional hermetic packaging that would endure in physiological environment. Lack of hermetic sealing likely poses a major obstacle in the chronic use of this system.

Between 2003 and 2004, acute stimulation with the IMI electrode array was tested in 20 subjects with advanced RP, of which 19 reported light perception. The visual percepts were reported in different shapes, sizes, colors, and brightness, even if only one electrode was activated (Hornig et al. 2007). The threshold charge measured from 15 patients fell within the safe limit of charge capacity of the iridium oxide electrodes (Keseru et al. 2012). The chronic performance of the device was evaluated in four subjects during a follow-up period of over 9 months, and the results showed that the implant did not cause tissue damage or abnormal cell growth in the eye. The patients were able to discriminate two stimulation points and recognize simple shapes when multiple electrodes were activated (Richard et al. 2007). Device performance beyond 9 months, however, is unclear. In 2016, Pixium Vision, which acquired and further developed IMI technology, launched a clinical trial to assess the safety and effectiveness of IRIS II, a 150-electrode epiretinal device, in ten patients with retinal dystrophy. Though the technical details of the IRIS II system are not publicized yet, several distinguishing features have been unveiled—a higher number of electrodes than the existing epiretinal systems, an explantable design that allows the electrode array to be safely removed and a smart camera that captures changes of the visual scene to avoid temporal redundancy that is common to the conventional frame-based image acquisition methods.

EPIRET3 is the latest retinal implant model from Epi-Ret. A prominent distinguishing feature of EPIRET3 is that the implant, apart from the external camera and the image processor, fits entirely within the eyeball, unlike the Argus and IMI implants that both have intraocular electrodes connected transclerally to extraocular electronics. This completely wireless design eliminates the need to suture any component on the outside of the eyeball. The array containing 25 protruding electrodes, each measured 100 μm in diameter and 25 μm in height, were attached to the macula by two tacks (Roessler et al. 2009; Klauke et al. 2011). These electrodes are manufactured from gold covered with a thin layer of iridium oxide. The entire implant is coated with parylene C to ensure biocompatibility and encapsulated by silicone to protect the electronics. Encapsulation of the device using a conformal layer of polymer enjoys the benefit of a compact size but typically has a shorter lifetime than hermetic packaging (Vanhoestenberghe and Donaldson 2013).

EPIRET3 was implanted in six RP patients in 2006 and removed 4 weeks later, according to the study design (Klauke et al. 2011). The stimulation thresholds were within the electrochemical safe limit for charge injection of the iridium oxide electrodes. The protruding electrodes may have lowered the thresholds by having improved contacts with the retina. The subjects were able to differentiate simple stimulation patterns, such as a circle or a line. A 2-year follow-up study in five subjects after the removal of the device indicate that, other than moderate gliosis at the tacks (which were left in place), no major structural disruption or alteration occurred in the eye (Menzel-Severing et al. 2012).

Subretinal Prostheses

Subretinal prostheses sit between the degenerated photoreceptor layer and the RPE. They pass current to the outer and middle sections of the retina (e.g., bipolar cells), therefore taking advantage of the existing neural processing in these retinal layers and meanwhile possibly avoiding the direct stimulation of ganglion cell axons that causes distortion of the visual perception (albeit retinal reorganization of the remaining retinal neurons may result in worse distortion of visual perceptions). The surgery to implant subretinal devices is considerably more difficult because of having to detach the retina and/or cut across the highly vascular choroid, and the limited subretinal space puts a constraint on the implant size, but it allows the implant to be held in place by pressure, without the need of a tack as is used for epiretinal prostheses, although subretinal implants may use a silicone oil tamponade (Stingl et al. 2013a) to guard against retinal detachment. Compared to epiretinal implantation where the vitreous flow and choroidal perfusion is unhindered, subretinal implantation may block the fluid communication between the retina and the choroid, obstructing heat dissipation from the retina and nutrient transport to the retina. Whether this could result in the atrophy of the retinal tissues around the implant area in the long term is under debate (Rizzo and Wyatt 1997; Peachey and Chow 1999; Sailer et al. 2007).

Two basic approaches to subretinal stimulation have been developed: one that uses a standard electrode array and the other that uses a microphotodiode array (MPDA). From the system perspective, the first approach is similar to the aforementioned epiretinal implants in the sense that images are acquired and processed by an external device and the electrode array only functions as a slave current source under the command of the stimulator chip. In contrast, MPDA itself detects light, eliminating the need for cameras as the visual scene is projected by the lens on the array. Each microphotodiode in the array functions independently by transforming local luminance level, in a proportional manner, into electrical pulses and directly stimulating the retinal neurons nearby. Since the MPDA is intraocularly located, patients enjoy the benefits of using eye movement, instead of head movement, to scan the visual scene.

Artificial silicon retina (ASR) from Optobionics, a Chicago-based company, is the first implant of this kind that entered clinical trials (Chow et al. 2004). The ASR microchip is a silicon-based device that contains approximately 5000 isolated microphotodiodes each bonded with a 9×9 μm iridium oxide electrode. This device is electrically passive, only driven by light. ASR was implanted in ten RP patients, and six of them had vision levels that allowed a follow-up of >7 years (Chow et al. 2010). The device was well tolerated, and visual function improvements were observed in most of the patients, however, mostly in areas far from the implant site (Chow et al. 2004, 2010). The investigators attributed the improvements to the neurotrophic effects of the implant that rescued or preserved the damaged retinal tissues, rather than the electrical activation of the neurons. Examination of the output current of these microphotodiodes revealed amplitude of several nA, far below the μA level needed for neuronal activation (Palanker et al. 2005), thus proving inadequate to drive meaningful prosthetic vision if solely relying on the incident light.

Technological variants that aim to provide enhanced photocurrents are instead pursued in the later MPDA devices.

Alpha-IMS, developed by Retina Implant AG in Germany, also uses a MPDA for light detection and current generation but includes externally powered circuits to amplify the photocurrents. Two forms of power supply to the circuits have been developed: wired and wireless. In the investigational device, power is supplied by a percutaneous cable that crosses the skin behind the ear, while in the commercial device (Alpha-IMS), the percutaneous cable is replaced by a subdermal power module for wireless transmission (Wilke et al. 2011; Stingl et al. 2013b). The MPDA chip consists of 1500 independently operating elements that each includes a light-sensitive photodiode connected to a differential amplifier, whose output is coupled to a square-shaped titanium nitride (TiN) electrode (50 × 50 μm). The chip has a size of 3 × 3 mm, estimated to cover a visual angle of 11° × 11° and a thickness of approximately 70 μm when placed on the polyimide foil. The investigational device has an additional 4 × 4 array of light insensitive TiN electrodes on the tip of the chip for direct stimulation independent from the photodiode outputs (Fig. 1.4a) (Zrenner et al. 2011; Wilke et al. 2011). It was found from the direct stimulation that the minimum charge transfer of a single electrode located at the subretinal space to generate visual percepts was typically between 20 and 60 nC per pulse (Zrenner et al. 2011).

The interim report of the clinical trial of Alpha-IMS, the wirelessly powered commercial version of the device, was recently published (Stingl et al. 2015). Since 2009, Alpha-IMS has been implanted in 29 patients with end-stage hereditary eye diseases: 25 with RP and 4 with cone-rod dystrophy. Within 12 months postoperative, 25 patients reported light perception and 21 showed significant improvements in the performance of visually guided daily living tasks, recognition tasks and mobility. Three patients were able to read some letters that subtended a visual angle between 5° and 10°. The spacing of 70 μm between each neighboring electrode offers a theoretical visual acuity of 20/250. Grating visual acuity measured from these patients roughly matched this theoretical limit, as the best grating acuity reported was 20/200. Not surprisingly, visual function outcome depends on foveal eccentricity—foveal placement of the device allows superior performance compared to the parafoveal and nonfoveal placement (Stingl et al. 2013c, 2015). The investigators noted a decrease of visual function over time in a number of patients, due to technical failure of the implants that usually occurred 3–12 months after the implantation, necessitating explanting the device. One problem common to the early devices was cable breakage that was caused by the mechanical stress on the intraorbital cable by eye movement. This problem was successfully solved by surgical introduction of a parabulbar loop that minimized the stress. Short lifetime of the hermetic seal is another major issue causing the device failure, as the corrosion of the chip gradually led to the loss of its function. According to the investigators, modified encapsulation technology has shown encouraging results in animal studies and is currently under assessment in the ongoing clinical trial (Stingl et al. 2013b, 2015;). However, long-term implantation success in patients still has not been achieved.

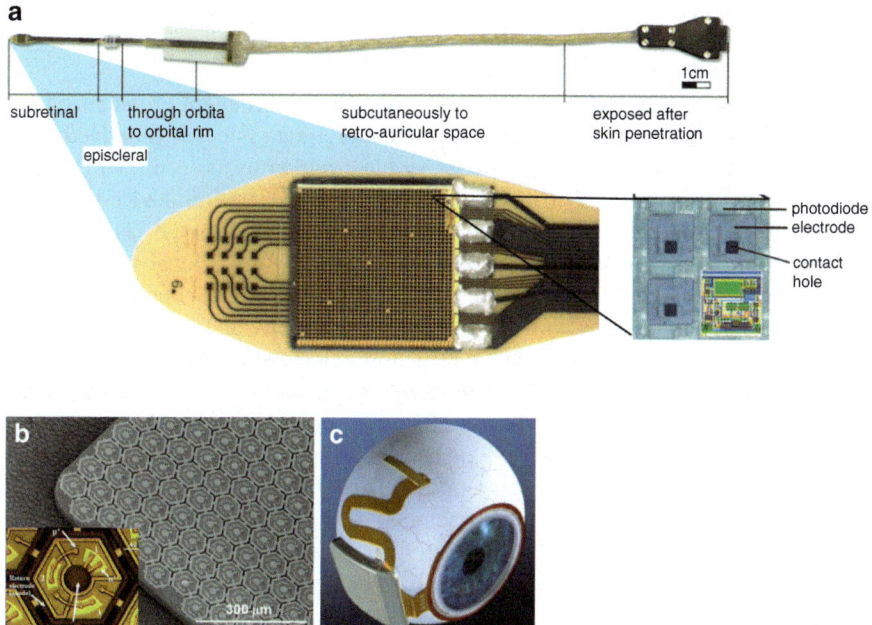

Fig. 1.4 Subretinal prostheses. (**a**) Prototype of the Alpha-IMS predecessor, an investigational device that includes 16 additional electrodes for direct stimulation. The overview of the implant (*top*) and the detailed view of the microphotodiode array (MPDA) with an additional 4 × 4 array of the TiN electrodes attached to the end (*bottom*). The MPDA chip consists of 1500 photodiodes on a surface area of 3 × 3 mm. Figure from Zrenner et al. (2011). (**b**) MPDA of the photovoltaic prosthesis developed by the Palanker group. *Inset*: Blown-up view of a single stimulating element with three photodiodes in series. Images from Wang, L., Mathieson, K., Kamins, T. I., Loudin, J. D., Galambos, L., Goetz, G., Sher, A., Mandel, Y., Huie, P., Lavinsky, D., Harris, J. S. & Palanker, D. V. 2012. Photovoltaic retinal prosthesis: implant fabrication and performance. *J Neural Eng*, 9, 046014. (**c**) IOP Publishing. Reproduced with permission. All rights reserved. (**c**) Prototype of the 256-channel Boston retinal implant. *Left*: Concept of the device with the secondary coil surrounding the cornea. *Right*: Electrodes bonded to the feedthrough of the hermetic case. Images from Kelly et al. (2011), with permission of Elsevier

Different from Alpha-IMS that relies on external power supply to amplify the stimulation currents, the photovoltaic retinal prosthesis developed by Palanker et al. (Palanker et al. 2005; Mathieson et al. 2012) offers an alternative that obviates the need for complex electrical circuitry and transscleral cabling. Instead of electrical amplification, this approach adopts optical amplification by converting ambient visual scene into high intensity near infrared (NIR, 880–915 nm) laser pulsing that is projected onto the subretinal photodiode array by a video goggle. The laser projection system increases the photocurrent by a factor of ~1000, theoretically sufficient to drive retinal neural stimulation. Importantly, the laser energy is within established safety margins. Each element in the photodiode array consists of a central iridium oxide electrode surrounded by two or three photodiodes in series to increase the dynamic range of the charge injection from the electrodes (Fig. 1.4b). This device has not yet entered clinical phase; therefore its safety and efficacy in human subjects are unknown.

The MIT-Harvard group that forms the Boston Retinal Implant Project is one of the earliest groups in retinal prosthesis. Their subretinal system was derived from the epiretinal design, and it uses a passive electrode array (i.e., no MPDA) for stimulation. The group has progressed from the first-generation device that contained 15 electrodes to a new generation 256-channel prototype. The marked increase in the number of electrodes presented substantial challenges to the electronic system and hermetic sealing. In order to drive 256 independently controlled channels, telemetry system with enhanced power capacity and higher data rate is desired. As shown in Fig. 1.4c, the investigators relocated the transceiver secondary coils from the temporal region of the eye to the anterior to allow for an increased size that improves inductive coupling efficiency with the external primary coils (Kelly et al. 2011, 2013). The prototype also features a novel design of high-count 256 ceramic feedthroughs in a titanium case (Fig. 1.4c, right), the hermeticity of which was evaluated to support a lifetime of 5–10 years, although a more definitive assessment warrants further testing in carefully controlled physiological environments (Shire et al. 2014; Kelly et al. 2013). This device is currently at the preclinical stage.

Suprachoroidal Prostheses

Suprachoroidal prostheses have electrodes placed between the choroid and the sclera. In comparison with the epiretinal and subretinal counterparts, suprachoroidal implants are relatively distant from the retina. This separation potentially reduces the risks of retinal damage from the surgery and the implant. Abundance of the blood vessels at the choroid makes the thermal dissipation of less concern as heat generated at the choroid layer should be carried away by the increased blood flow (Parver et al. 1983; Hadjinicolaou et al. 2015). But on the other hand, with lengthened current travel path from the electrode to the target tissue, this stimulation site may be disadvantaged by the elevated perceptual threshold and worsened spatial resolution (Yamauchi et al. 2005). To better steer the current flow through the retina, a return electrode is typically located in the anterior part of the eye, for example, inside the vitreous cavity or on the cornea, to be less invasive.

Semichronic suprachoroid transscleral (STS) prosthesis (Fig. 1.5a) developed by Fujikado et al. in Japan was tested in two RP patients in 2011 (Fujikado et al. 2011). The electronic metal case was placed subdermal behind the ears and the implant in a scleral pocket (6 × 5 mm) formed by cutting a flap in the sclera (Morimoto et al. 2011). The stimulation chip contained an array of 49 platinum electrodes (500 μm diameter), among which 9 were active. Only four to six out of these nine electrodes were able to elicit phosphenes within the current limit, and the charge levels were considerably higher than those reported with the epiretinal implants. Nonetheless, it

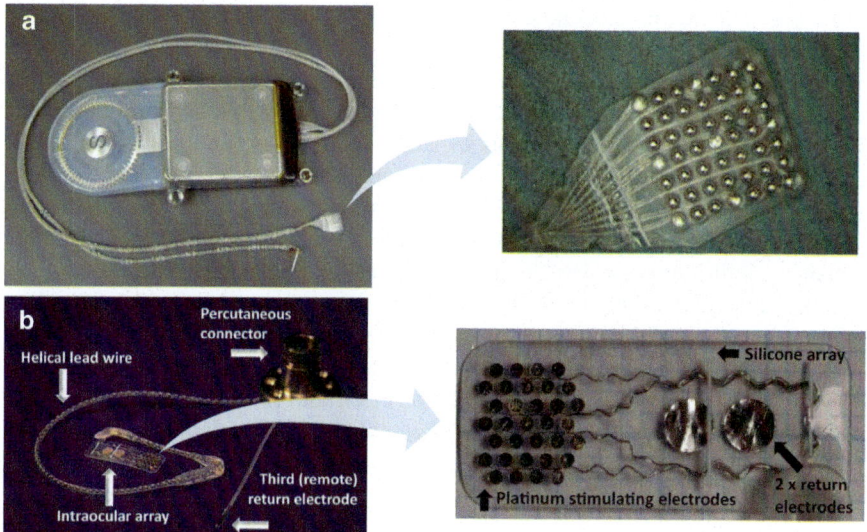

Fig. 1.5 Suprachoroidal prostheses. (**a**) The STS implant including the suprachoroidal stimulating array and the remote return electrode. *Inset*: The exploded view of the stimulating array containing 49 electrodes. Images reprinted from Fujikado et al. (2011). (**b**) The BVA implant with one remote return and two other return electrodes on the suprachoroidal array. *Inset*: The exploded view of the implant chip consisting of 33 platinum stimulating electrodes and two large return electrodes on the silicone substrate. Images adapted from Ayton et al. (2014)

allows the patients to localize objects and reach for them better than the chance level. Neither retinal detachment nor hemorrhage was observed after the surgeries. The device was removed 4 weeks after implantation so long-term information is not available.

Bionic Vision Australia (BVA) Consortium, a joint team of researchers from different Australian research institutes, is developing several prototypes simultaneously with the aim to achieve wide-view suprachoroidal prosthetic vision and high-resolution epiretinal prosthetic vision. From 2012 to 2014, their early suprachoroidal prototype was tested in three RP patients in a Phase I clinical trial. The intraocular array, inserted in the scleral pocket, consists of 33 platinum stimulating electrodes (400 and 600 μm diameter) and 2 large return electrodes (2000 μm diameter) on silicone substrate (Fig. 1.5b). The 13 stimulating electrodes on the outer ring were shorted together to form a large common ground. In addition, a third electrode was implanted subcutaneously behind the ear, serving as an extraocular return (Ayton et al. 2014; Shivdasani et al. 2014). Thus the implant contains a total of 20 individually addressable stimulating electrodes and 4 optional returns. The intraocular electrode array is connected by a helical lead wire to a percutaneous plug behind the ear. The plug, similar to what has been used in cochlear implants, serves as an exposed connector to the external control, allowing direct and flexible stimulation without the need for complex electronics and telemetry in this early prototype. The investigators noted that, in future devices, the plug will be replaced by wireless communication systems.

Postsurgical monitoring up to 2 years indicates that the implant remains stable and functional in the suprachoroidal space without causing significant retinal edema or atrophy. Phosphenes were reliably evoked in all three patients below the charge density of 158 $\mu C/cm^2$ for 600 μm electrodes and 237 $\mu C/cm^2$ for 400 μm electrode (Ayton et al. 2014), within the safe limit for chronic stimulation of platinum electrodes (350 $\mu C/cm^2$). The threshold was found to be dependent on retina-electrode distance, similar to what was reported on epiretinal implants (De Balthasar et al. 2008). An increase of the threshold was observed over time along with an increase in the measure of the retina-electrode distance, but the cause is unclear. Various return configurations were tested, showing higher efficacy with monopolar pattern (one large return distant from the stimulating electrode) (Shivdasani et al. 2014). In visual function tests, all three patients were able to localize light spots markedly better than the chance level, and one patient achieved an estimated Landolt C visual acuity of 2.62longMAR (20/8397) (Ayton et al. 2014).

Summary

From LeRoy's experiment in 1775 to Brindley and Lewin prosthesis in 1969 to the present Argus II and Alpha-IMS systems that are approved for the clinical treatment of RP, electrical stimulation of the human visual system has progressed a long way from intellectual curiosity to reality. Built upon the early proof-of-concept work, the field of retinal prostheses entered the fast track in the 1990s. The most recent two decades witnessed the tremendous advancement not only in the development of the prosthetic systems but also in the understanding of the electrical retinal stimulation. A variety of the devices, implanted at the different retinal locations, have been put into preclinical and clinical testing. Electrode characteristics and the key clinical results of the aforementioned bioelectronic retinal prosthetic systems are summarized in Table 1.1.

A majority of these devices that reached the clinical phase have been demonstrated to restore useful artificial vision in patients blinded for years from outer retinal degeneration. The vision restored, though still is limited compared with what a normally sighted person sees, enables the patients to perform visually guided tasks such as object recognition and mobility. Yet physiological and technical challenges remain, limiting the visual experience of the subjects. To best mimic the normal vision in prosthesis patients, new strategies that could add on to the existing prosthesis framework have been pursued, primarily in the following directions: (1) improving the visual acuity, (2) increasing the visual field, (3) enhancing stimulation selectivity, (4) substituting head movement with eye movement for visual field scanning, and (5) incorporating a retinal encoder in stimulation to better account for the visual processing. It is in the foreseeable future that with the continued advancement in material science, electronics, and microfabrication, facilitated by further

Table 1.1 Comparison of the bioelectronic stimulation systems in electrodes and clinical outcomes

Location	Device	Electrode		Size (μm)	Pitch (μm)	Power/ data link	Clinical results				Reference
		Material	Count				Number of subjects	Implant duration	Visual acuity	Visual field	
Epi.	Argus I	Pt	16	250, 500	800	RF	6	11 years and ongoing	20/3244 VGA	10° × 10°	Caspi et al. (2009) Yue et al. (2015)
	Argus II	Pt	60	200	525	RF	30	8 years and ongoing	20/1262 VGA	19° × 111°	Humayun et al. (2012) Ho et al. (2015)
	IMI	IrOx	49	50, 100 200, 360	N/A	RF, IR	20 (A) 4 (C)	3 months (A) 9 months (C)	N/A	N/A	Hornig et al. (2007) Richard et al. (2007)
	EPIRET3	IrOx	25	100	500	RF (IOC)	6	4 weeks	N/A	N/A	Roessler et al. (2009) Klauke et al. (2011)
Sub.	Alpha-IMS	TiN	1500	50	70	MPDA, RF	29	6 years and ongoing	20/200 VGA 20/546 LCA	10° × 10°	Stingl et al. (2013b) Stingl et al. (2015)
	Photovoltaic prosthesis	IrOx	N/A	20, 40	75, 145	MPDA, IR	N/A	N/A	N/A	N/A	Mathieson et al. (2012) Lorach et al. (2015)
	Boston implant	IrOx	256	N/A	N/A	RF	N/A	N/A	N/A	N/A	Kelly et al. (2013)
Supra.	STS	Pt	49 (9 active)	500	700	RF	2	4 weeks	N/A	20° × 16°	Fujikado et al. (2011)
	BVA	Pt	33	400, 600	1000	Wired	3	3 years and going	20/4451 LCA	12° × 12°	Ayton et al. (2014)

Abbreviations: *Epi.* epiretinal, *Sub.* subretinal, *Supra.* suprachoroidal, *Pt* platinum, *IrOx* iridium oxide, *TiN* titanium nitride, *IOC* intraocular coil, *A* acute, *C* chronic, *VGA* visual grating acuity, *LCA* Landolt C acuity. The photovoltaic prosthesis and Boston implant have not entered the clinical phase understanding of the retinal signal processing, prosthetic vision that better mimics normal visual percepts will become reality, benefiting millions of blind patients worldwide.

Compliance with Ethical Requirements Lan Yue declares no conflict of interest. James D. Weiland holds patents with Second Sight Medical Products, Inc., Sylmar, CA. Mark S. Humayun has commercial interest and hold patents with Second Sight Medical Products, Inc., Sylmar, CA. No human or animal studies were carried out by the authors for this article.

References

Ayton LN, Blamey PJ, Guymer RH, Luu CD, Nayagam DA, Sinclair NC, Shivdasani MN, Yeoh J, Mccombe MF, Briggs RJ, Opie NL, Villalobos J, Dimitrov PN, Varsamidis M, Petoe MA, Mccarthy CD, Walker JG, Barnes N, Burkitt AN, Williams CE, Shepherd RK, Allen PJ, Consortium BVAR. First-in-human trial of a novel suprachoroidal retinal prosthesis. PLoS One. 2014;9:e115239.

Beck H, Boden WE, Patibandla S, Kireyev D, Gutpa V, Campagna F, Cain ME, Marine JE. 50th Anniversary of the first successful permanent pacemaker implantation in the United States: historical review and future directions. Am J Cardiol. 2010;106:810–8.

Beltran WA, Cideciyan AV, Lewin AS, Iwabe S, Khanna H, Sumaroka A, Chiodo VA, Fajardo DS, Roman AJ, Deng WT, Swider M, Aleman TS, Boye SL, Genini S, Swaroop A, Hauswirth WW, Jacobson SG, Aguirre GD. Gene therapy rescues photoreceptor blindness in dogs and paves the way for treating human X-linked retinitis pigmentosa. Proc Natl Acad Sci U S A. 2012;109:2132–7.

Bressler NM. Age-related macular degeneration is the leading cause of blindness. JAMA. 2004;291:1900–1.

Brindley GS, Lewin W. The sensations produced by electrical stimulation of the visual cortex. J Neurophysiol. 1968;196:479–93.

Brummer S, Turner M. Electrical stimulation of the nervous system: the principle of safe charge injection with noble metal electrodes. Bioelectrochem Bioenerg. 1975;2:13–25.

Busskamp V, Duebel J, Balya D, Fradot M, Viney TJ, Siegert S, Groner AC, Cabuy E, Forster V, Seeliger M, Biel M, Humphries P, Paques M, Mohand-Said S, Trono D, Deisseroth K, Sahel JA, Picaud S, Roska B. Genetic reactivation of cone photoreceptors restores visual responses in retinitis pigmentosa. Science. 2010;329:413–7.

Caspi A, Dorn JD, Mcclure KH, Humayun MS, Greenberg RJ, Mcmahon MJ. Feasibility study of a retinal prosthesis: spatial vision with a 16-electrode implant. Arch Ophthalmol. 2009;127:398–401.

Chow AY, Chow VY, Packo KH, Pollack JS, Peyman GA, Schuchard R. The artificial silicon retina microchip for the treatment of vision loss from retinitis pigmentosa. Arch Ophthalmol. 2004;122:460–9.

Chow AY, Bittner AK, Pardue MT. The artificial silicon retina in retinitis pigmentosa patients (an American Ophthalmological Association thesis). Trans Am Ophthalmol Soc. 2010;108:120–54.

Curcio CA, Owsley C, Jackson GR. Spare the rods, save the cones in aging and age-related maculopathy. Invest Ophthalmol Vis Sci. 2000;41:2015–8.

De Balthasar C, Patel S, Roy A, Freda R, Greenwald S, Horsager A, Mahadevappa M, Yanai D, Mcmahon MJ, Humayun MS, Greenberg RJ, Weiland JD, Fine I. Factors affecting perceptual thresholds in epiretinal prostheses. Invest Ophthalmol Vis Sci. 2008;49:2303–14.

Den Hollander AI, Ten Brink JB, De Kok YJ, Van Soest S, Van Den Born LI, Van Driel MA, Van De Pol DJ, Payne AM, Bhattacharya SS, Kellner U, Hoyng CB, Westerveld A, Brunner HG,

Bleeker-Wagemakers EM, Deutman AF, Heckenlively JR, Cremers FP, Bergen AA. Mutations in a human homologue of Drosophila crumbs cause retinitis pigmentosa (RP12). Nat Genet. 1999;23:217–21.

Dobelle WH, Mladejovsky M, Girvin J. Artificial vision for the blind: electrical stimulation of visual cortex offers hope for a functional prosthesis. Science. 1974;183:440–4.

Dowling J. Current and future prospects for optoelectronic retinal prostheses. Eye (Lond). 2009;23:1999–2005.

Fariss RN, Li ZY, Milam AH. Abnormalities in rod photoreceptors, amacrine cells, and horizontal cells in human retinas with retinitis pigmentosa. Am J Ophthalmol. 2000;129:215–23.

Foerster BO. zur Pathophysiologie der Sehbahn und der Sehsphare. J Psychol Neurol Lpz. 1929;39:463–85.

Friedman DS, O'Colmain BJ, Munoz B, Tomany SC, McCarty C, de Jong PT, Nemesure B, Mitchell P, Kempen J, Eye Diseases Prevalence Research G. Prevalence of age-related macular degeneration in the United States. Arch Ophthalmol. 2004;122:564–72.

Fujikado T, Kamei M, Sakaguchi H, Kanda H, Morimoto T, Ikuno Y, Nishida K, Kishima H, Maruo T, Konoma K, Ozawa M, Nishida K. Testing of semichronically implanted retinal prosthesis by suprachoroidal-transretinal stimulation in patients with retinitis pigmentosa. Invest Ophthalmol Vis Sci. 2011;52:4726–33.

Hadjinicolaou AE, Meffin H, Maturana MI, Cloherty SL, Ibbotson MR. Prosthetic vision: devices, patient outcomes and retinal research. Clin Exp Optom. 2015;98:395–410.

Hartong DT, Berson EL, Dryja TP. Retinitis pigmentosa. Lancet. 2006;368:1795–809.

Heier JS, Brown DM, Chong V, Korobelnik JF, Kaiser PK, Nguyen QD, Kirchhof B, Ho A, Ogura Y, Yancopoulos GD, Stahl N, Vitti R, Berliner AJ, Soo Y, Anderesi M, Groetzbach G, Sommerauer B, Sandbrink R, Simader C, Schmidt-Erfurth U, Groups VS. Intravitreal aflibercept (VEGF trap-eye) in wet age-related macular degeneration. Ophthalmology. 2012;119:2537–48.

Ho AC, Humayun MS, Dorn JD, da Cruz L, Dagnelie G, Handa J, Barale PO, Sahel JA, Stanga PE, Hafezi F, Safran AB, Salzmann J, Santos A, Birch D, Spencer R, Cideciyan AV, de Juan E, Duncan JL, Eliott D, Fawzi A, Olmos de Koo LC, Brown GC, Haller JA, Regillo CD, del Priore LV, Arditi A, Geruschat DR, Greenberg RJ, Group AIS. Long-term results from an epiretinal prosthesis to restore sight to the blind. Ophthalmology. 2015;122:1547–54.

Hornig R, Zehnder T, Velikay-Parel M, Laube T, Feucht M, Richard G. The IMI retinal implant system. Artificial sight. New York: Springer; 2007.

Horsager A, Greenwald SH, Weiland JD, Humayun MS, Greenberg RJ, Mcmahon MJ, Boynton GM, Fine I. Predicting visual sensitivity in retinal prosthesis patients. Invest Ophthalmol Vis Sci. 2009;50:1483–91.

Humayun MS, Prince M, De Juan E Jr, Barron Y, Moskowitz M, Klock IB, Milam AH. Morphometric analysis of the extramacular retina from postmortem eyes with retinitis pigmentosa. Invest Ophthalmol Vis Sci. 1999;40:143–8.

Humayun MS, Dorn JD, da Cruz L, Dagnelie G, Sahel JA, Stanga PE, Cideciyan AV, Duncan JL, Eliott D, Filley E, Ho AC, Santos A, Safran AB, Arditi A, Del Priore LV, Greenberg RJ, Group AIS. Interim results from the international trial of second sight's visual prosthesis. Ophthalmology. 2012;119:779–88.

Jackson GR, Owsley C, Curcio CA. Photoreceptor degeneration and dysfunction in aging and age-related maculopathy. Ageing Res Rev. 2002;1:381–96.

Kelly SK, Shire DB, Chen J, Doyle P, Gingerich MD, Cogan SF, Drohan WA, Behan S, Theogarajan L, Wyatt JL, Rizzo JF III. A hermetic wireless subretinal neurostimulator for vision prostheses. IEEE Trans Biomed Eng. 2011;58:3197–205.

Kelly SK, Shire DB, Chen J, Gingerich MD, Cogan SF, Drohan W, Ellersick W, Krishnan A, Behan S, Wyatt JL, Rizzo JF. Developments on the Boston 256-channel retinal implant. In: IEEE international conference on multimedia and expo workshops (ICMEW): IEEE; 2013. p. 1–6.

Keseru M, Feucht M, Bornfeld N, Laube T, Walter P, Rossler G, Velikay-Parel M, Hornig R, Richard G. Acute electrical stimulation of the human retina with an epiretinal electrode array. Acta Ophthalmol. 2012;90:e1–8.

Kim SY, Sadda S, Pearlman J, Humayun MS, De Juan E Jr, Melia BM, Green WR. Morphometric analysis of the macula in eyes with disciform age-related macular degeneration. Retina. 2002;22:471–7.

Klauke S, Goertz M, Rein S, Hoehl D, Thomas U, Eckhorn R, Bremmer F, Wachtler T. Stimulation with a wireless intraocular epiretinal implant elicits visual percepts in blind humans. Invest Ophthalmol Vis Sci. 2011;52:449–55.

Krause F, Schum H. Die epileptischen Erkrankungen. Neue Deutsche Chirurgie. 1931;49:482–6.

Kringelbach ML, Jenkinson N, Owen SL, Aziz TZ. Translational principles of deep brain stimulation. Nat Rev Neurosci. 2007;8:623–35.

Lilly JC, Austin GM, Chambers WW. Threshold movements produced by excitation of cerebral cortex and efferent fibers with some parametric regions of rectangular current pulses (cats and monkeys). J Neurophysiol. 1952;15:319–41.

Lilly JC, Hughes JR, Alvord EC Jr, Galkin TW. Brief, noninjurious electric waveform for stimulation of the brain. Science. 1955;121:468–9.

Lorach H, Goetz G, Mandel Y, Lei X, Galambos L, Kamins TI, Mathieson K, Huie P, Dalal R, Harris JS, Palanker D. Performance of photovoltaic arrays in-vivo and characteristics of prosthetic vision in animals with retinal degeneration. Vis. Res. 2015;111, 142e148.

Mahadevappa M, Weiland JD, Yanai D, Fine I, Greenberg RJ, Humayun MS. Perceptual thresholds and electrode impedance in three retinal prosthesis subjects. IEEE Trans Neural Syst Rehabil Eng. 2005;13:201–6.

Marc RE, Jones BW, Watt CB, Strettoi E. Neural remodeling in retinal degeneration. Prog Retin Eye Res. 2003;22:607–55.

Mathieson K, Loudin J, Goetz G, Huie P, Wang L, Kamins TI, Galambos L, Smith R, Harris JS, Sher A, Palanker D. Photovoltaic retinal prosthesis with high pixel density. Nat Photonics. 2012;6:391–7.

Medeiros NE, Curcio CA. Preservation of ganglion cell layer neurons in age-related macular degeneration. Invest Ophthalmol Vis Sci. 2001;42:795–803.

Menzel-Severing J, Laube T, Brockmann C, Bornfeld N, Mokwa W, Mazinani B, Walter P, Roessler G. Implantation and explantation of an active epiretinal visual prosthesis: 2-year follow-up data from the EPIRET3 prospective clinical trial. Eye (Lond). 2012;26:501–9.

Morimoto T, Kamei M, Nishida K, Sakaguchi H, Kanda H, Ikuno Y, Kishima H, Maruo T, Konoma K, Ozawa M, Nishida K, Fujikado T. Chronic implantation of newly developed suprachoroidal-transretinal stimulation prosthesis in dogs. Invest Ophthalmol Vis Sci. 2011;52:6785–92.

Nanduri D, Fine I, Horsager A, Boynton GM, Humayun MS, Greenberg RJ, Weiland JD. Frequency and amplitude modulation have different effects on the percepts elicited by retinal stimulation. Invest Ophthalmol Vis Sci. 2012;53:205.

Niparko JK. Cochlear implants: principles & practices. Philadelphia, PA: Lippincott Williams & Wilkins; 2009.

Opie NL, Burkitt AN, Meffin H, Grayden DB. Heating of the eye by a retinal prosthesis: modeling, cadaver and in vivo study. IEEE Trans Biomed Eng. 2012;59:339–45.

Palanker D, Vankov A, Huie P, Baccus S. Design of a high-resolution optoelectronic retinal prosthesis. J Neural Eng. 2005;2:S105–20.

Parver LM, Auker CR, Carpenter DO. Choroidal blood flow. III. Reflexive control in human eyes. Arch Ophthalmol. 1983;101:1604–6.

Peachey NS, Chow AY. Subretinal implantation of semiconductor-based photodiodes: progress and challenges. J Rehabil Res Dev. 1999;36:371–6.

Pezaris JS, Eskandar EN. Getting signals into the brain: visual prosthetics through thalamic microstimulation. Neurosurg Focus. 2009;27:E6.

Potts A, Inoue J. The electrically evoked response (EER) of the visual system. II. Effect of adaptation and retinitis pigmentosa. Investig Ophthalmol. 1969;8:605.

Rakoczy EP, Lai CM, Magno AL, Wikstrom ME, French MA, Pierce CM, Schwartz SD, Blumenkranz MS, Chalberg TW, Degli-Esposti MA, Constable IJ. Gene therapy with recombinant adeno-associated vectors for neovascular age-related macular degeneration: 1 year follow-up of a phase 1 randomised clinical trial. Lancet. 2015;386:2395–403.

Richard G, Hornig R, Keserü M, Feucht M. Chronic epiretinal chip implant in blind patients with retinitis pigmentosa: long-term clinical results. Invest Ophthalmol Vis Sci. 2007;48:666.

Richer S, Stiles W, Statkute L, Pulido J, Frankowski J, Rudy D, Pei K, Tsipursky M, Nyland J. Double-masked, placebo-controlled, randomized trial of lutein and antioxidant supplementation in the intervention of atrophic age-related macular degeneration: the Veterans LAST study (Lutein Antioxidant Supplementation Trial). Optometry. 2004;75:216–30.

Rizzo JF, Wyatt J. Review: prospects for a visual prosthesis. Neuroscientist. 1997;3:251–62.

Rizzo JF 3rd, Wyatt J, Loewenstein J, Kelly S, Shire D. Perceptual efficacy of electrical stimulation of human retina with a microelectrode array during short-term surgical trials. Invest Ophthalmol Vis Sci. 2003;44:5362–9.

Roessler G, Laube T, Brockmann C, Kirschkamp T, Mazinani B, Goertz M, Koch C, Krisch I, Sellhaus B, Trieu HK, Weis J, Bornfeld N, Rothgen H, Messner A, Mokwa W, Walter P. Implantation and explantation of a wireless epiretinal retina implant device: observations during the EPIRET3 prospective clinical trial. Invest Ophthalmol Vis Sci. 2009;50:3003–8.

Sailer H, Shinoda K, Blatsios G, Kohler K, Bondzio L, Zrenner E, Gekeler F. Investigation of thermal effects of infrared lasers on the rabbit retina: a study in the course of development of an active subretinal prosthesis. Graefes Arch Clin Exp Ophthalmol. 2007;245:1169–78.

Santos A, Humayun MS, De Juan E Jr, Greenburg RJ, Marsh MJ, Klock IB, Milam AH. Preservation of the inner retina in retinitis pigmentosa. A morphometric analysis. Arch Ophthalmol. 1997;115:511–5.

Shire DB, Jones WK, Karbasi A, Behan S, Gingerich M, Kelly S, Wyatt JL, Rizzo JF. Advanced hermetic feedthrough and packaging technology for the Boston retinal prosthesis. Invest Ophthalmol Vis Sci. 2014;55:1835.

Shivdasani MN, Sinclair NC, Dimitrov PN, Varsamidis M, Ayton LN, Luu CD, Perera T, Mcdermott HJ, Blamey PJ. Factors affecting perceptual thresholds in a suprachoroidal retinal prosthesis factors affecting retinal prosthesis thresholds. Invest Ophthalmol Vis Sci. 2014;55:6467–81.

Stingl K, Bach M, Bartz-Schmidt KU, Braun A, Bruckmann A, Gekeler F, Greppmaier U, Hortdorfer G, Kusnyerik A, Peters T, Wilhelm B, Wilke R, Zrenner E. Safety and efficacy of subretinal visual implants in humans: methodological aspects. Clin Exp Optom. 2013a;96:4–13.

Stingl K, Bartz-Schmidt KU, Besch D, Braun A, Bruckmann A, Gekeler F, Greppmaier U, Hipp S, Hortdorfer G, Kernstock C, Koitschev A, Kusnyerik A, Sachs H, Schatz A, Stingl KT, Peters T, Wilhelm B, Zrenner E. Artificial vision with wirelessly powered subretinal electronic implant alpha-IMS. Proc Biol Sci. 2013b;280:20130077.

Stingl K, Bartz-Schmidt KU, Gekeler F, Kusnyerik A, Sachs H, Zrenner E. Functional outcome in subretinal electronic implants depends on foveal eccentricity. Invest Ophthalmol Vis Sci. 2013c;54:7658–65.

Stingl K, Bartz-Schmidt KU, Besch D, Chee CK, Cottriall CL, Gekeler F, Groppe M, Jackson TL, Maclaren RE, Koitschev A, Kusnyerik A, Neffendorf J, Nemeth J, Naeem MAN, Peters T, Ramsden JD, Sachs H, Simpson A, Mandeep SS, Wilhelm B, Wong D, Zrenner E. Subretinal visual implant alpha IMS–clinical trial interim report. Vis Res. 2015;111:149–60.

Tsai D, Chen S, Protti DA, Morley JW, Suaning GJ, Lovell NH. Responses of retinal ganglion cells to extracellular electrical stimulation, from single cell to population: model-based analysis. PLoS One. 2012;7:e53357.

Van Balken MR, Vergunst H, Bemelmans BL. The use of electrical devices for the treatment of bladder dysfunction: a review of methods. J Neurol. 2004;172:846–51.

Vanhoestenberghe A, Donaldson N. Corrosion of silicon integrated circuits and lifetime predictions in implantable electronic devices. J Neural Eng. 2013;10:031002.

Veraart C, Raftopoulos C, Mortimer JT, Delbeke J, Pins D, Michaux G, Vanlierde A, Parrini S, Wanet-Defalque M-C. Visual sensations produced by optic nerve stimulation using an implanted self-sizing spiral cuff electrode. Brain Res. 1998;813:181–6.

Wang L, Mathieson K, Kamins TI, Loudin JD, Galambos L, Goetz G, Sher A, Mandel Y, Huie P, Lavinsky D, Harris JS, Palanker DV. Photovoltaic retinal prosthesis: implant fabrication and performance. J Neural Eng. 2012;9:046014.

Weiland JD, Humayun MS. Visual prosthesis. Proc IEEE. 2008;96:1076–84.

Weiland JD, Cho AK, Humayun MS. Retinal prostheses: current clinical results and future needs. Ophthalmology. 2011;118:2227–37.

Weitz AC, Behrend MR, Ahuja AK, Christopher P, Wei J, Wuyyuru V, Patel U, Greenberg RJ, Humayun MS, Chow RH. Interphase gap as a means to reduce electrical stimulation thresholds for epiretinal prostheses. J Neural Eng. 2014;11:016007.

Weitz AC, Nanduri D, Behrend MR, Gonzalez-Calle A, Greenberg RJ, Humayun MS, Chow RH, Weiland JD. Improving the spatial resolution of epiretinal implants by increasing stimulus pulse duration. Sci Transl Med. 2015;7:318ra203.

Wells J, Wroblewski J, Keen J, Inglehearn C, Jubb C, Eckstein A, Jay M, Arden G, Bhattacharya S, Fitzke F. Mutations in the human retinal degeneration slow (RDS) gene can cause either retinitis pigmentosa or macular dystrophy. Retinal degeneration. New York: Springer; 1993.

Wilke R, Gabel VP, Sachs H, Bartz Schmidt KU, Gekeler F, Besch D, Szurman P, Stett A, Wilhelm B, Peters T, Harscher A, Greppmaier U, Kibbel S, Benav H, Bruckmann A, Stingl K, Kusnyerik A, Zrenner E. Spatial resolution and perception of patterns mediated by a subretinal 16-electrode array in patients blinded by hereditary retinal dystrophies. Invest Ophthalmol Vis Sci. 2011;52:5995–6003.

Wong IY, Poon MW, Pang RT, Lian Q, Wong D. Promises of stem cell therapy for retinal degenerative diseases. Graefes Arch Clin Exp Ophthalmol. 2011;249:1439–48.

Wood AJ, Fine SL, Berger JW, Maguire MG, Ho AC. Age-related macular degeneration. N Engl J Med. 2000;342:483–92.

Yamauchi Y, Franco LM, Jackson DJ, Naber JF, Ziv RO, Rizzo JF, Kaplan HJ, Enzmann V. Comparison of electrically evoked cortical potential thresholds generated with subretinal or suprachoroidal placement of a microelectrode array in the rabbit. J Neural Eng. 2005;2:S48–56.

Yue L, Falabella P, Christopher P, Wuyyuru V, Dorn J, Schor P, Greenberg RJ, Weiland JD, Humayun MS. Ten-year follow-up of a blind patient chronically implanted with epiretinal prosthesis Argus I. Ophthalmology. 2015;122:2545–2552.e2541.

Zrenner E, Bartz-Schmidt KU, Benav H, Besch D, Bruckmann A, Gabel VP, Gekeler F, Greppmaier U, Harscher A, Kibbel S, Koch J, Kusnyerik A, Peters T, Stingl K, Sachs H, Stett A, Szurman P, Wilhelm B, Wilke R. Subretinal electronic chips allow blind patients to read letters and combine them to words. Proc Biol Sci. 2011;278:1489–97.

Chapter 2
Retinal Prostheses: Bioengineering Considerations

Yao-Chuan Chang, James D. Weiland, and Mark S. Humayun

Engineering Challenges

Several retinal prostheses have been tested in clinical trials, and two systems have regulatory approval, but many technical challenges need to be resolved to enable a long-lasting, high-resolution device. Microelectronics cannot survive long-term exposure to water and ions inside the body; thus, new materials or processes are required for forming thin and robust isolation barriers to protect the electronics. To support the increased number of electrodes, more efficient electronic circuits with safe levels of power consumption are needed for parallel stimulation of 100s of individual contacts. The electrode array, as the main interface between implant and retina, can be improved from many aspects. The electrode material must support higher charge density due to the reduction of electrode size and safety concerns with current materials. To improve the attachment as well as alleviate damage, the electrode substrates need to be flexible for close fit to the curvature of the retina. In addition, electrical stimulation patterns can be further optimized for ideal visual perception and power consumption reduction. Finally, the usage of state-of-the-art camera technology and

Y.-C. Chang, Ph.D. (✉)
Department of Biomedical Engineering, University of Southern California,
Los Angeles, CA 90089, USA
e-mail: yaochuac@usc.edu

J.D. Weiland, Ph.D. (✉)
Department of Biomedical Engineering, University of Southern California,
Los Angeles, CA 90089, USA

USC Roski Eye Institute, Institute for Biomedical Therapeutics, University of Southern California, Los Angeles, CA 90033, USA
e-mail: weiland@umich.edu

M.S. Humayun, M.D., Ph.D.
Roski Eye Institute, Institute for Biomedical Therapeutics,
University of Southern California, Los Angeles, CA 90033, USA
e-mail: humayun@med.usc.edu

© Springer International Publishing AG 2018
M.S. Humayun, L.C. Olmos de Koo (eds.), *Retinal Prosthesis*, Essentials in Ophthalmology, https://doi.org/10.1007/978-3-319-67260-1_2

advanced algorithms for video processing has great potential to compensate for the limited visual task performance shown by patients using lower-resolution devices.

Packaging

Perhaps the most important technology for any medical implant is the hermetic packaging. This requires a set of materials to be used to form a barrier that is virtually impervious to penetration by water or ions. Since a perfect barrier for an infinitely long time is not possible, instead leak rate specifications are developed based on empirical and theoretical models; too detailed to review here, but see Vanhoestenberghe and Donaldson (2013) and Jiang and Zhou (2010). These specifications ensure that a high percentage (greater than 99%) of implanted devices will last for decades in the body. Generally, encapsulation and hermetic enclosure are two commonly used methods that were described by Donaldson (Vanhoestenberghe and Donaldson 2013) (Fig. 2.1).

Encapsulation

Encapsulation relies on using a conformal layer of material(s) to coat the electronics (Fig. 2.1: *Top*). Metals and ceramics are the best water barriers, but depositing thin films of these materials in a conformal manner is technically challenging. Polymers, such as silicone, can be applied conformally but have poor water vapor transmission rates (i.e., water vapor readily passes through silicone). However, good protection can be achieved if the polymer coating is tightly fit to the surface of the electronics;

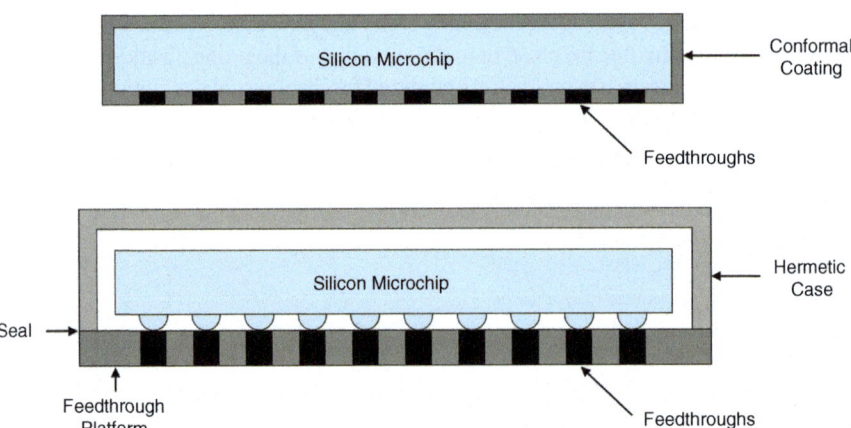

Fig. 2.1 Hermetic packaging schemes. *Top*: Encapsulation - Encapsulating the entire electronic chip with conformal coating provide an ideal protection scheme, but to date no coating technology has proven adequate for long-term implantation. *Bottom*: Enclosure - An electronics module is placed inside an enclosure, which includes a feedthrough platform with conductors and a case or lid. The feedthrough and case are sealed together

water cannot condense on the surface after penetrating the polymers. One of the drawbacks of this strategy is the requirement for a level of surface cleanliness which is extremely difficult to achieve in practice (Vanhoestenberghe and Donaldson 2013). If the chip surface is not free of particulates or if there is the presence of voids in the conformal coating, then water can condense at these imperfections and ultimately lead to failure of electronics. As evidence, some reports show that the retinal prosthesis devices encapsulated with polymers can survive only for 1–2 years, thus suggesting process development must be improved before encapsulation become a viable approach.

Most of the current research on improving the performance of encapsulation focuses on replacing polymer-based film with different materials. A multilayer, multi-material film composed of both diamond-like coating and metal films has been proposed as an alternative to polymer coatings (Weiland et al. 2013). The structure demonstrates robust ion barrier properties and good conformality around the corner and edge of the coating, though long-term testing has not been completed. Ultra-nano-crystalline diamond film has also been used to form an inert and thin coating layer; however, a better dielectric material might be needed to embed into the layer due to the insufficient insulating ability at high voltage (Xiao et al. 2006). Recently, amorphous silicon carbide (a-SiCx:H or a-SiC) has been used by several groups, due to its excellent dielectric property, resistance to degradation, and capability of deposition when fabricating (Cogan et al. 2003; Sharma et al. 2012). However, the deposition rate for SiC is relatively slow (0.2–0.5 µm/h) at low temperature (<400 °C), and the compressive stress of a-SiC intrinsic (0.2–0.3 GPa) might limit the maximum film thickness (<5 µm) to guarantee good adhesion and prevent from device distortion. In summary, thin-film encapsulants remain a research topic that has tremendous potential, but no clear solution at this time.

Enclosure

Hermetic enclosures demonstrate relatively robust performance; thus, almost all clinically approved implantable neurostimulation devices adopt this approach. Traditionally, the titanium or ceramic cases (like a shell) are accompanied by a feedthrough (a substrate with isolated conductors channeling the electrical signals across enclosure); combined, the case and feedthrough form a complete enclosure (Jiang and Zhou 2010) (Fig. 2.1: *Bottom*). However, compared with the enclosed electronics, case thickness and feedthrough conductor spacing (pitch) enlarge the size of implants significantly. For example, the Argus II uses this style of packaging, and the implant size is determined largely by the size requirement for the feedthrough substrate that has 60 independent stimulus channels. The Argus II hermetic enclosure represents a great engineering accomplishment, specifically a 10× reduction in volume and 3× increase in independent channels, compared with the previous state of the art, which was the cochlear implant. Yet, contrast the dimensions of the feedthrough features (100s of microns), with the minimum size of other electronic components used in implants (integrated circuit pads can be made 50 μm diameter, electrodes can have features below 10 μm, and integrated transistor sizes are less than 0.1 μm), and it is clear that a packaging technology defines the size of the implant, and relatively large available technology limits further size reduction of the Argus II and other implants that use enclosures. Functionally, the number of channels will be limited, thereby limiting the best possibly visual acuity. Additionally, the present size does occasionally lead to conjunctival erosion, which may occur less with a smaller implant. Therefore, improving hermetic packaging technology is critical for both improving resolution and increasing biocompatibility.

Advanced processing techniques for enclosures have been developed to increase the density of conducting channels. Suaning et al. proposed a method that places patterned platinum foil to form lines between two alumina sheets (a ceramic commonly used in medical implants) with gaps filled with alumina particles suspended in viscous liquid (Suaning et al. 2006). Subsequent high-temperature operation promotes crystal growth in alumina, thus fusing the sheets. To connect with the internal electronics, holes corresponding to the bond pads are drilled through one of the alumina sheets. Schuettler et al. achieved 360 channels in a feedthrough with dimension less than 25 mm² by a screen printing approach (Schuettler et al. 2010). Another group fabricated high-density feedthrough with a stack of alumina layer and platinum wire in interlocking pattern (Gill et al. 2013) (Fig. 2.2). With proper heat temperature operation and compression, the transverse cutting section normal to the wires results in a patterned grid of platinum conductors in order, with helium leak rate less than 8×10^{-11} mbar-l/s, which is generally considered an acceptable leak rate, though this must also consider the implant volume.

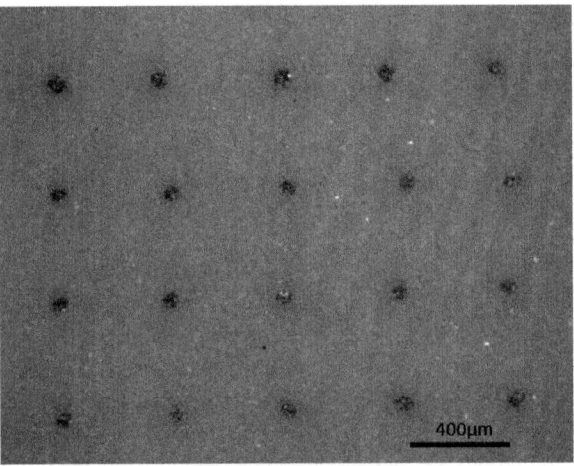

Fig. 2.2 High-density feedthrough technology. Front view shows a patterned grid of platinum conductors embedded in alumina substrate. Image from Gill et al. (2013)

Electronics Module

The electronics used for retinal prostheses are varied and encompass several sub-specialties of electrical engineering. The connection between the camera and the electrode array constitutes a signal chain. The most complex signal chains involves the following steps: (1) conversion of video data into digital data format; (2) processing of the digital camera data to convert brightness detected in a particular region into a level of stimulation to be applied to the retina; (3) encoding of the stimulation levels for all electrodes into a serial data stream; (4) generation of a wireless, radio frequency transmission signal that carries both power and the serial data stream to the implant; (5) RF energy transmission between a pair of well-aligned inductive coils, one external and one implanted; (6) power recovery and data decoding from the received RF signal; and (7) generation of stimulation pulses based on the camera input. Steps 1–4 are done in a wearable external system, steps 6 and 7 are done in the implant, and step 5 links the two. The signal chain can be simplified, in some ways, by placing the light-sensing element inside the eye, which will eliminate some of the steps above, but add complexity to the implant design, which in this case must have electronics for photon detection as well as stimulus current generation.

For those systems using an external camera, both camera and supporting hardware do not represent significant technical challenges. Rapid advances in cell phone camera quality and miniaturization benefit the external system by making available camera hardware that meets the specifications in terms of pixel density. In contrast, greater design challenges remain for the wireless transfer of data and power and for the design of efficient stimulator electronics. Reviews of these areas are listed below.

Telemetry

Wireless transmission of data and power has been adopted for most retinal prosthetic systems, due to the requirement for small size and continuously refreshed data. Devices that operate on batteries, such as deep brain stimulators, are implanted in the upper trunk and thus have room to accommodate batteries, whereas the orbit is space constrained. Retinal implants must be constantly fed with the latest camera data, so a wireless data link is required. Deep brain stimulators run on preset stimulation parameters and only update data during a clinic visit using special external programming hardware.

Since the wireless power and data transmission has the potential to interfere, design of retinal prostheses should consider power and data together. However, a fundamental conflict exists when choosing the optimal wireless transmission frequency. Data and power are often transmitted using the same radio frequency signal. Data is encoded by modulating the amplitude or phase of signals. The implant electronics recovers both power and data from this signal, for implant operation. For advanced retinal prosthesies, the data rate should be on the order of megabits/sec and the carrier frequency to reliably support such a data rate is typically set to an order of magnitude higher, say 10 MHz (Zhou et al. 2008). Yet, to maintain the power transmission efficiency, the frequency needs to be set under 10 MHz due to signal attenuation across tissue and internal AC-DC conversion (Wang et al. 2006).

Multiband transmitters which separate the frequencies for power and data individually have been regarded as one of the most effective approaches for retinal prosthesis RF transmission. In this approach, different transmitter and receiver coils were designed and embedded in the device for power and data links (Chen et al. 2013). The power signal requires larger coils and operates at lower frequency for efficient power transmission, whereas the data signal can be transmitted through smaller coils at higher frequency, since the data signal demands lower power. Although the efficiency can be dramatically improved, such a system requires careful design to prevent interference or cross talk between the links. Previous study has shown that a 256-channel retinal prosthesis system with dual band telemetry can be realized on the bench top, thus indicating that the technique might be feasible in a clinical device (Chen et al. 2013).

Optical transmission of both power and data has also been studied for other retinal implants. For a subretinal prosthesis, a optobionic microphotodiode array was proposed to directly convert incident light to electric power, but the generated power is not sufficient to activate neurons on the retina (Palanker et al. 2005). The other optical application was presented by Gross et al. who combined the infrared optical data link with inductive power link (Gross et al. 1999). This design was ultimately included in the IMI epiretinal prosthesis. The optical data link can achieve a data rate of 200 Kb/s.

Integrated Circuit

Depending on the type of retinal implants, generally, the integrated circuit (IC) needs to perform multiple functions, including AC-DC conversion (if using inductive power), data demodulation (if using wireless data transmission), digital control, analog voltage or current stimulus, and reverse telemetry (from the implant to an external system) for diagnostic information about the implant. Among them, the design of voltage drivers is challenging since both positive and negative voltages are needed for supplying adequate anodic and cathodic current for charge balanced stimulation. The size and power consumption are other competing requirement for the stimulator chip.

Liu et al. have designed, fabricated, and tested several generations of multichannel stimulator IC for retinal prostheses. The most recent contribution of the group is to completely embed the data demodulation, timing controlled rectification (power efficient AC-DC conversion), digital control, and 256-channel independent stimulus drivers into a compact system (Chen et al. 2010) (Fig. 2.3). In particular, the timing-controlled rectifier eliminates a great amount of power loss, when compared to a typical diode-based rectifier, during AC-DC conversion. IC area is reduced with the

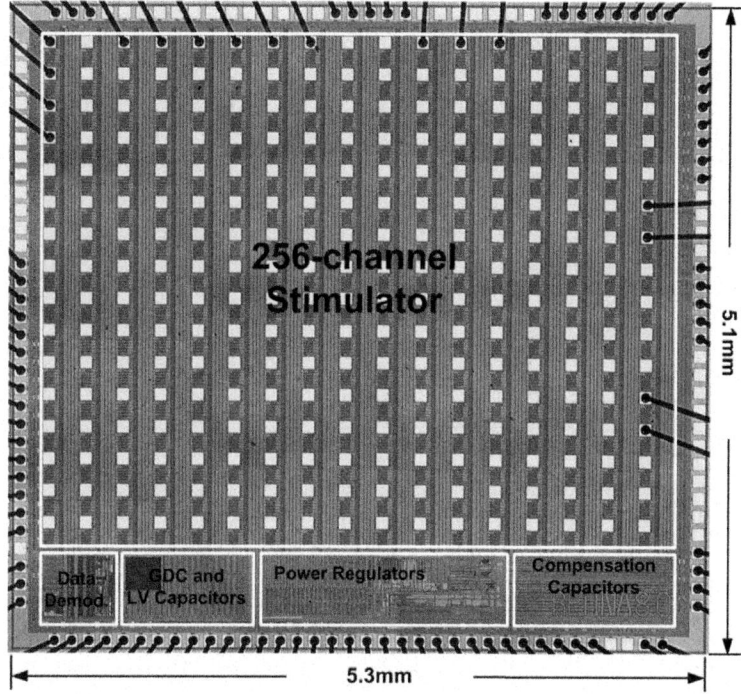

Fig. 2.3 Chip microphotograph of the 256-channel epiretinal stimulator manufactured by Liu and colleagues. The chip has integrated power conditioning and data decode, and 256 independent output channels. (Image from Chen et al. 2010 with permission from IEEE)

advance of circuit-under-pad layout which utilizes multiple metal layers in the process to place bond pads over the circuitry. This platform was validated as functional in a benchtop end-to-end system validation (Chen et al. 2013), with real-time visual feedback and wireless power/data links (Fig. 2.4).

Ortmanns and colleagues have created a 232-channel stimulator chip which was manufactured in 0.35 μm CMOS fabrication (Ortmanns et al. 2006). The overall size of the chip is less than 5 × 5 mm, and its high-voltage feature allows high stimulus current through small electrodes. They also constructed a charge-balancing scheme to balance the current sources without the need for large capacitors on every output, thus reducing the accumulated charge on electrodes which might ultimately results in neural injury and saving space on the overall implant size. The balance pulse will be triggered when recorded electrode voltages between pulses exceed ±50 mV.

A chip with 256 channels has been developed in 0.18 μm CMOS, as part of a subretinal prosthesis (Shire et al. 2012). Similar to other epiretinal applications, the chip contains power/data telemetry modules and reverse low-rate data link for monitoring the electrode voltage on any output and transmission. This chip is not designed to reside underneath the retina; rather the proposed system uses a

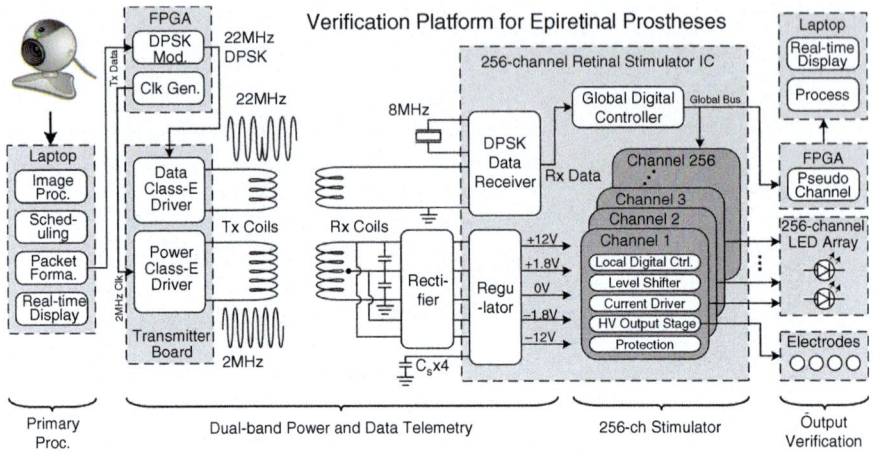

Fig. 2.4 The exemplary system diagram of the verification platform for epiretinal prostheses with multiband approaches. (Reproduced from Chen et al. 2013, with permission of IEEE)

microelectrode array as a retinal interface. The drivers are designed with high-voltage components allowing of a wide range of stimulus current and can be configured as sources or sinks arbitrarily for current steering.

Another retinal stimulator with 96 channels has been designed for allowing current steering between local sources and sinks which presumably can facilitate focused stimulation to the intended site (Dommel et al. 2009). The voltage drivers of this chip are implemented by specific high-voltage transistors which are fabricated in 0.35 μm process, whereas the remaining chip features are operated with low-voltage transistors for space and power saving. For localized stimulus, the chip contains special switch design that allows any electrode to be configured as either a center current source or within a group of six surrounding sinks forming a hexagonal pattern near the source. This concept has been tested on a test chip which accommodates 14 hexagonal electrode mosaic with switching and two current drivers. The other feature of this chip is to short all electrodes for dissipating accumulated charge during the intermediate period between stimuli. This is another approach to ensure charge balance without the need for large capacitors on each output.

A high-density 512-channel retinal stimulator chip has been developed for supporting higher-resolution retinal prostheses (Monge et al. 2013). A novel feature of this chip is autocalibration circuitry on the output, which can be used to improve stimulation precision and eliminate charge accumulation. The use of 65 nm transistors in the design allows an increase in output channels as well as a reduction in chip size to 4.5×3.1 mm^2, which has the potential to be installed entirely inside the eye if proper packaging techniques are used. The whole chip is operated at ± 2.5 V to reduce power consumption. However, with this choice of a low voltage supply, the output current range might be limited.

Electrode

With the advance of retinal prostheses, such as the Argus II and Alpha-IMS, electrode technology, especially in term of fabrication, has been improved significantly for implantable bioelectronics. Conventional implants, such as deep brain stimulator cochlear implants, only require handmade electrode assemblies, featuring several platinum contacts supported by a polymer substrate. In contrast, due to the requirement for a comparatively high number of densely spaced contacts, to match the 2D retinal structure, photolithography and micromachining techniques have been used to fabricate these arrays. In addition to using advanced manufacturing techniques, the electrode materials have been improved to compensate for limited electrode size and allow adequate charge injection capability. Argus II and Alpha-IMS take advantage of state-of-the-art platinum gray and titanium nitride, respectively. Both are superior to bulk platinum, which is typically used for neurostimulation. Compared with 0.1–0.35 mC/cm^2 charge injection capability for platinum (Rose and Robblee 1990), the platinum gray and titanium nitride have pushed the limits to 1 and 0.9 mC/cm^2 (Zhou et al. 2013; Weiland et al. 2002). The electrode array substrate serves to hold in place the electrodes. Since this serves as a mechanical interface with the retina, care must be taken to avoid a design that will damage the retina, which is a very delicate tissue. Most devices use polymer substrates that have an integrated cable and lead to connect the electronics with the electrode array. In contrast, the Alpha-IMS has electrodes patterned directly on the silicon IC. This has the advantage of avoiding complex routing schemes to connect the electronics and the array, but the silicon IC is rigid compared to a polymer array, and can potentially damage the retina.

Visual field and acuity is another fundamental problem facing retinal prostheses. The structure of human retina is a roughly 2.5 cm diameter hemisphere attaching to the back of the eye, spanning approximately 60° nasal and superior field, about 70° inferior field, as well as 90° temporal field (Barton and Benatar 2003). To completely cover the entire retina, an electrode array with $\pi * (d/2)^2$ or almost 5 cm^2 dimension is required. For an epiretinal prosthesis, the array size is mostly limited by the incision that can be safely made in the implant surgery (less than 5 mm). A wide-field foldable array that can be inserted through a 5 mm eye incision has been proposed by Ameri et al. (2009). This approach can potentially provide a visual field of 34° once it expands in eye, compared with 19° for Argus II and 11° for Alpha-IMS. Based on this concept, subsequent development has been tested through long-term implantation in animal eyes to validate its feasibility (Zhang et al. 2013). On the other hand, subretinal implant size is mainly limited by the risk of retinal detachment attributed to the insertion of an array underneath the retina. With the increase of subretinal array size, a higher risk of detaching the entire retina can be expected. Retinal detachment has disastrous and irreversible consequences for retina health, so the surgery process for the subretinal implant Alpha-IMS includes a silicone oil injection to mitigate the likelihood of retinal detachment (Stingl et al. 2013).

Visual acuity is used to measure the spatial resolution of a visual system. For people with normal visual acuity (20/20 vision), two points separated by 1 arcmin, equivalent to 4.5 μm of retina, can be resolved. Based on this finding, the electrode pitch (the distance between the centers of two adjacent electrodes), size, and electrode-retina contact would contribute the perception of retinal implant users. The best reported visual grating acuities for Argus II and Alpha-IMS user are 20/1260 and 20/546, respectively, which roughly matches the theoretical limits of electrode spacing (525 and 70 μm) (Yue et al. 2016). Practically, since a threshold amount of charge is required to create a perception of light, the electrode size cannot be selected arbitrary small (since the amount of safe charge is reduced with electrode area). The contact between retina tissue and electrode is another factor for acuity, since the retina, along with the surrounding physiological vitreous, can be regarded as inhomogeneous conductive medium. The vitreous (or saline after vitrectomy) is more conductive than the retina and underlying tissue. Thus, there exists the scenario that stimulus current, from an electrode away from the retina, preferentially passes through the vitreous, parallel to the retina, and disperses current significantly. Special recessed electrodes have been developed for constraining the electric field or increasing selectivity (Suesserman et al. 1991; Wilke et al. 2011). For the subretinally implanted recessed 3D electrode, the bipolar cell has further been found to migrate into the cavity of electrode, thus inducing a more selective and robust neural interface although device removal would be more complicated (Butterwick et al. 2009; Djilas et al. 2011) (Fig. 2.5). Some groups use localized return electrodes near the stimulating electrode to confine the stimulus current and achieve focal activation of neurons (Palanker et al. 2005). Recently, Habib et al. (2013) tested the performance of a hexagonal electrode array that has one stimulating electrode surrounded by six "guard" (return) electrodes through a whole mount rabbit retina model. The results show that the difference of RGC thresholds inside and outside of the hex guards can be enlarged to twofold higher, implying the ability for localized stimulation (Habib et al. 2013). However, since the proximity between stimulating and return electrode caused current shunting through more conductive saline rather than retina, the required current threshold is elevated as the stimulation efficiency declines compared with simple monopolar configuration (which uses a distant return electrode and forces current to pass through the retina).

Electrical Stimulation

Various electrical stimulation strategies have been used to improve the performance of visual perception from different perspectives. Theoretically, since visual perception is determined by the types of activated neurons, selective electrical stimulation of specific neurons can change the actual perception. Moreover, since about 20 different circuit network mosaics in the retina have been identified for extracting distinct visual information (Dacey 1999), the stimulation patterns that can produce firing patterns specific to each mosaic have been investigated to generate more

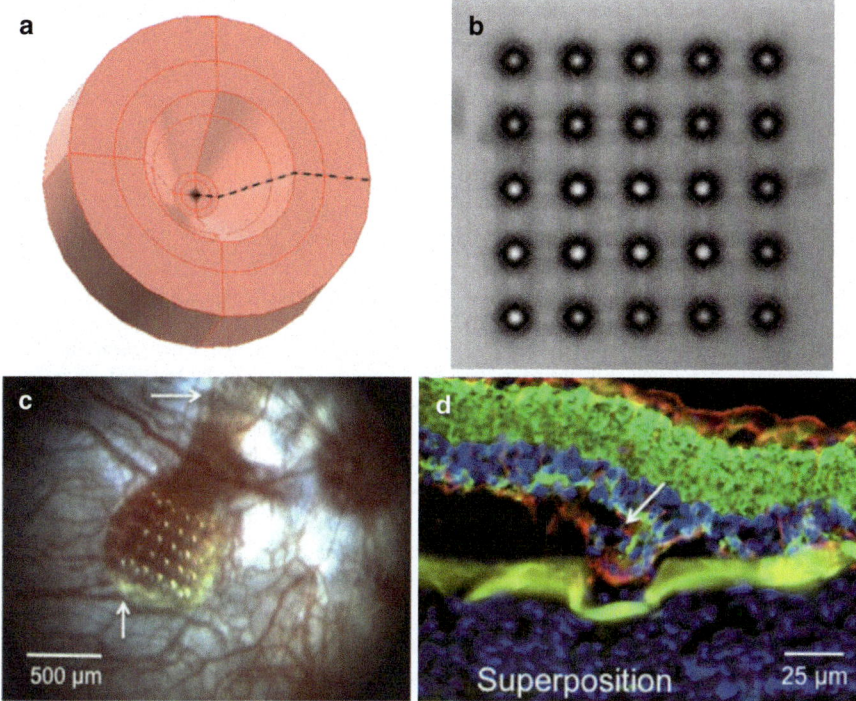

Fig. 2.5 Example of a recessed 3D electrode, array and its implant performance. (**a**) Geometries of a 3D recessed electrode. (**b**) A fabricated electrode array. (**c**) The endoscopic control of the subretinal implant position. (**d**) Neuronal integration of the P23H rat retina in a 3D retinal implant well. Blue DAPI nuclear staining shows the cell nuclei integrating the well. Red GFAP immunolabeling shows the absence of a major retinal gliosis at the site of integration in retinal implant well. Green Goα immunolabeling visualizes ON bipolar cells integrated into the implant well (*arrow*).

natural input to the visual cortex. The stimulation efficiency has been also addressed to manipulate the threshold of neurons or alleviate phosphene fading in response to continuous stimulation.

Selective Stimulation

The final output of the retina is retinal ganglion cells (RGCs) that collectively transmit preprocessed visual information to the brain, and those neurons are the main targets for retinal prosthetic research since the visual percepts are mostly determined by their activation patterns. The RGC neurons can be activated directly by sufficient depolarization of the RGC membrane or indirectly via synaptic transmission from activated bipolar cells (BP). Studies have shown that RGCs are more easily excited by short duration pulse (<150 μs), whereas BPs tend to respond preferentially to longer pulse width (Margalit and Thoreson 2006; Fried et al. 2006;

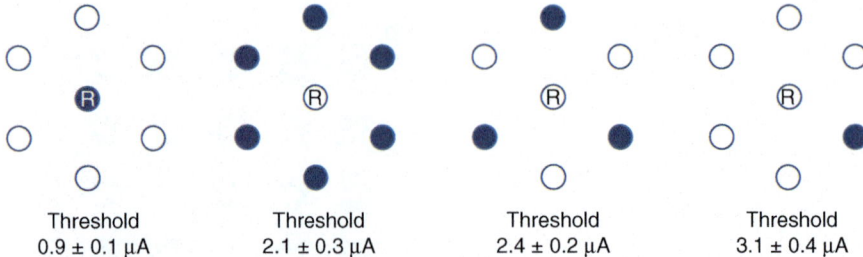

Fig. 2.6 Spike thresholds for several stimulation configurations. Region adjacent to the center recording electrode (R) on the hexagonal array is shown, with filled circles indicating active electrodes for stimulation and open circles denoting unused electrodes. All active electrodes were simultaneously stimulated at the same current amplitude. In addition to the standard setup (*left*), three alternative configurations were tested: all neighboring electrodes, three electrodes, and a single neighboring electrode. Threshold currents are shown as averages over eight cells and indicate lowest value found when multiple electrode combinations were tested. Corresponding charge densities were 0.09, 0.22, 0.25, and 0.32 mC/cm². Electrodes were 60 μm apart. (The figure is redrawn and reproduced from Sekirnjak et al. (2006), with permission from the American Physiological Society)

Freeman et al. 2010). For ideal retinal implants, each electrode should only activate nearby RGCs, thus forming small round visual percepts. However, precious clinical study for patients with Argus II epiretinal implants reported most evoked percepts by single electrode were elongated and aligned with the estimated axon paths in the retina, suggesting the activation of axon bundles (Nanduri et al. 2011, 2012). A similar phenomenon has also been validated through electrically elicited responses in salamander and rodent model using calcium imaging techniques (Behrend et al. 2009; Weitz et al. 2013). To prevent streak-like perceptions, longer duration pulse has been used to produce more confining retinal responses to the site of the electrode through indirect stimulation (Freeman et al. 2010). Chichilnisky et al. demonstrate that the manipulation of spatial patterns of current injection generated by high-density multielectrode can be used to selectively evoke action potential firing from individual ganglion cells, thus increasing the spatial resolution of stimulation (Sekirnjak et al. 2006; Jepson et al. 2013) (Fig. 2.6). In subretinal stimulation, the anodic-leading current pulse has been shown to result in differential thresholds for ON and OFF cells which might further be applied on targeted stimulation of ON/OFF signaling pathways (Jensen and Rizzo 2006).

Stimulation Encoding

In addition to targeting a specific cell type, any electrical stimulation protocol that seeks to create a more natural visual signal must recreate the typical spatiotemporal response. Ideally, such an approach could manipulate perception in terms of luminance, contrast, shape, color, and motion. Electrophysiological studies have shown that the response of RGCs can be predicted through a linear-nonlinear (*LN*) cascade model with a difference-of-Gaussians or wavelet-shaped characteristic spatial profile (Frishman et al. 1987; Meister and Berry 1999; Van Rullen and Thorpe 2001). Based on that idea, Bomash et al. have developed an adaptable *LN* model for a wide range of stimuli to more precisely investigate population encoding (Bomash et al. 2013). Eckmiller et al. proposed an encoder which models receptive field properties of primate RGCs as individual spatiotemporal filters (Eckmiller et al. 2005). For each filter, the parameters were trained through machine learning algorithms iteratively supervised with subject feedback to mimic the retinal information processing. The visual inputs from an asynchronous contrast sensor was also used for reconstructing the spatiotemporal properties of several RGC groups and possibly outperforms the frame-based inputs in term of temporal precision (Lorach et al. 2012). Recently, involuntary eye movements including microsaccades, drifts, and tremor were incorporated in retinal models. The result showed that the visual sensitivity to both spatial and temporal changes in luminance can be ameliorated (Olmedo-Payá et al. 2015). Yet, none of above conceptualized methods has been successfully applied on real retinal prostheses mainly due to the constraints on the electrode size. It is not yet possible to control single RGC or bipolar cells with a retinal prosthesis, which is necessary for the biological models to be effective.

Stimulation Efficiency

A more pertinent concern for clinical retinal implants is stimulus efficiency. Using lower stimulus intensity can extend the battery life of the external system (which supplies power for the implant). For the epiretinal implant Argus II, adding an interphase gap between the symmetric cathodic-first biphasic pulses or altering the stimulus to asymmetric anodic-first pulse with unbalanced duration can effectively reduce the required electrical stimulation thresholds (Weitz et al. 2014; Chang and Weiland 2016). Perceptions fade when high stimulus rates are used, but if stimulation pulses are applied at too low a rate, the percept will flicker and be less useful. For subretinal Alpha-IMS implants, the working frequency for stimulation is typically set to 5–20 Hz, and some patients claim that the lower frequency option helps in alleviating phosphene fading (Stingl et al. 2015). Another fading-resistant strategies proposed by Freeman and Fried include interleaving longer duration desensitizing pulses (1 ms) between the short duration (200 µs) stimulating pulse trains delivered as a function of incoming luminance (Freeman and Fried 2011). The desensitizing pulses are proposed to diminish the synaptically mediated response which is believed to cause desensitization, thus allowing luminance-driven pulse to elicit one to two spikes per pulse through direct activation of RGC. Until now, this strategy has not been experimentally validated.

Cameras and Video Processing

State-of-the-art cell phone cameras have vastly superior resolution compared with the retinal implant electrode array; therefore, little engineering research is needed on camera technology, except for incorporating depth information to aid in detection of important obstacles. However, since the visual perception integrates not only the signal from the retina but also the motion of eye/head and proprioception, camera positioning becomes a critical issue for prosthesis user to obtain a more natural perception. Video processing algorithms have potential to improve the performance of retinal prostheses through selectively highlighting important areas (nearby objects) and attenuating irrelevant background scene (far in distance).

Camera Positioning

The Alpha-IMS has imaging capability positioned underneath the retina. The electrically-evoked vision, eye and head coordinates naturally since the imaging components are located inside the eye thus move along with the eye. In contrast, the cameras of epiretinal implants are usually externally installed on a glasses frame, so head movement is needed to refresh an image. Although no controlled comparison has been studied in patients, the head-mounted camera seems to be less instinctive, and long-term training may be required for adaptation.

Novel Camera and Video Processing

The potential of depth cameras has been generally validated in the computer vision field and in commercial products such as the Microsoft Kinect. Some studies have extended this technology to the retinal prosthesis with conferring the ability to capture the relative distance between user and objects. McCarthy et al. has established a visual representation that augments intensity of regions of the current scene, based on the local variation of surface originated from the RGB and depth information (Mccarthy et al. 2013). Their results show that potentially important obstacles such as a low wall near a sidewalk in a scene can be accentuated and presented in the simulated prosthetic vision paradigm. Moreover, the depth information can be used as input to simultaneous localization and mapping (*SLAM*) algorithms which construct a map of an unknown environment while simultaneously keeping track of the location of user (Pradeep et al. 2009). This concept might ultimately be transformed into guidance cues to help retinal prosthesis users to pass through a complicated environment.

For epiretinal implants, a camera that can directly replace the role of the crystalline lens might be a solution for more natural vision. Nasiatka et al. have proposed an intraocular camera that can be implanted in the position of the crystalline lens (Nasiatka et al. 2010). Due to the limitation of space, a small cylindrical hermetic capsule about 3 mm in diameter and 4 mm long was designed to fit in the place, and an aspherical lens with extremely short back focal length (~1 mm) was used to form image on the wide dynamic rage CMOS sensor. With the power and control circuit behind the sensors, the visual information can be delivered to the stimulation chip, further driving the related stimulation patterns on the electrode array. Simulation of the intraocular camera experiment suggests that with the control ability of eye movement, the user can perform visual tasks in a more natural manner (Weiland and Humayun 2014).

Summary

Developments from different engineering perspectives have made significant advances and improved the performance of retinal implants, but much work still remains to achieve long-lasting, high-resolution device. Hermetic packaging has been developed to meet the standards for regulatory approval, but an ideal coating with both low-dimensional requirement and high durability is still not yet available. Electronics module have achieved complexity that is adequate for most of current systems, though more sophisticated designs are required for high transmission rate, low power consumption, as well as efficient and safe stimulus drivers. Electrode arrays now can be fabricated with requisite site density; however, more adaptable substrates with high flexibility are needed to ensure each electrodes form close contact with retina. Electrical stimulation strategies have been shown to alter the responses of retinal cells; therefore, better control over shape perception and stimulation efficiency can be expected with the advanced stimulation strategies.

Compliance with Ethical Requirements Yao-Chuan Chang declares no conflict of interest. James D. Weiland holds patents with Second Sight Medical Products, Inc., Sylmar, CA. Mark S. Humayun has commercial interest and hold patents with Second Sight Medical Products, Inc., Sylmar, CA. No human or animal studies were carried out by the authors for this article.

References

Ameri H, Ratanapakorn T, Ufer S, Eckhardt H, Humayun MS, Weiland JD. Toward a wide-field retinal prosthesis. J Neural Eng. 2009;6:035002.

Barton JJS, Benatar M. An introduction to perimetry and the normal visual field. In: Field of vision: a manual and atlas of perimetry. Totowa, NJ: Humana Press; 2003.

Behrend MR, Ahuja AK, Humayun MS, Weiland JD, Chow RH. Selective labeling of retinal ganglion cells with calcium indicators by retrograde loading in vitro. J Neurosci Methods. 2009;179:166–72.

Bomash I, Roudi Y, Nirenberg S. A virtual retina for studying population coding. PLoS One. 2013;8:e53363.

Butterwick A, Huie P, Jones BW, Marc RE, Marmor M, Palanker D. Effect of shape and coating of a subretinal prosthesis on its integration with the retina. Exp Eye Res. 2009;88:22–9.

Chang Y-C, Weiland JD. Threshold manipulation of retinal ganglion cells using precondition anodic stimulation. San Diego: Society of Neuroscience; 2016.

Chen K, Yang Z, Hoang L, Weiland J, Humayun M, Liu W. An integrated 256-channel epiretinal prosthesis. IEEE J Solid State Circuits. 2010;45:1946–56.

Chen K, Lo YK, Yang Z, Weiland JD, Humayun MS, Liu W. A system verification platform for high-density epiretinal prostheses. IEEE Trans Biomed Circuits Syst. 2013;7:326–37.

Cogan SF, Edell DJ, Guzelian AA, Ping Liu Y, Edell R. Plasma-enhanced chemical vapor deposited silicon carbide as an implantable dielectric coating. J Biomed Mater Res A. 2003;67:856–67.

Dacey DM. Primate retina: cell types, circuits and color opponency. Prog Retin Eye Res. 1999;18:737–63.

Djilas M, Oles C, Lorach H, Bendali A, Degardin J, Dubus E, Lissorgues-Bazin G, Rousseau L, Benosman R, Ieng SH, Joucla S, Yvert B, Bergonzo P, Sahel J, Picaud S. Three-dimensional electrode arrays for retinal prostheses: modeling, geometry optimization and experimental validation. J Neural Eng. 2011;8:046020.

Dommel NB, Wong YT, Lehmann T, Dodds CW, Lovell NH, Suaning GJ. A CMOS retinal neurostimulator capable of focussed, simultaneous stimulation. J Neural Eng. 2009;6:035006.

Eckmiller R, Neumann D, Baruth O. Tunable retina encoders for retina implants: why and how. J Neural Eng. 2005;2:S91–S104.

Freeman DK, Fried SI. Multiple components of ganglion cell desensitization in response to prosthetic stimulation. J Neural Eng. 2011;8:016008.

Freeman DK, Eddington DK, Rizzo JF 3rd, Fried SI. Selective activation of neuronal targets with sinusoidal electric stimulation. J Neurophysiol. 2010;104:2778–91.

Fried SI, Hsueh HA, Werblin FS. A method for generating precise temporal patterns of retinal spiking using prosthetic stimulation. J Neurophysiol. 2006;95:970–8.

Frishman LJ, Freeman AW, Troy JB, Schweitzer-Tong DE, Enroth-Cugell C. Spatiotemporal frequency responses of cat retinal ganglion cells. J Gen Physiol. 1987;89:599–628.

Gill EC, Antalek J, Kimock FM, Nasiatka PJ, Mcintosh BP, Tanguay ARJ, Weiland JD. High-density feedthrough technology for hermetic biomedical micropackaging. MRS Online Proc Libr Arch. 2013;1572:mrss13-1572-ss05-08. (6 pages)

Gross M, Buss R, Kohler K, Schaub J, Jager D. Optical signal and energy transmission for a retina implant. In: Engineering in Medicine and Biology, 1999. 21st annual conference and the 1999 annual fall meeting of the Biomedical Engineering Society. BMES/EMBS conference, 1999. Proceedings of the first joint 1999, 476, vol. 1.

Habib AG, Cameron MA, Suaning GJ, Lovell NH, Morley JW. Spatially restricted electrical activation of retinal ganglion cells in the rabbit retina by hexapolar electrode return configuration. J Neural Eng. 2013;10:036013.

Jensen RJ, Rizzo JF 3rd. Thresholds for activation of rabbit retinal ganglion cells with a subretinal electrode. Exp Eye Res. 2006;83:367–73.

Jepson LH, Hottowy P, Mathieson K, Gunning DE, Dabrowski W, Litke AM, Chichilnisky EJ. Focal electrical stimulation of major ganglion cell types in the primate retina for the design of visual prostheses. J Neurosci. 2013;33:7194–205.

Jiang G, Zhou DD. Technology advances and challenges in hermetic packaging for implantable medical devices. In: Zhou DD, Greenbaum E, editors. Implantable neural prostheses 2. New York: Springer; 2010.

Lorach H, Benosman R, Marre O, Ieng SH, Sahel JA, Picaud S. Artificial retina: the multichannel processing of the mammalian retina achieved with a neuromorphic asynchronous light acquisition device. J Neural Eng. 2012;9:066004.

Margalit E, Thoreson WB. Inner retinal mechanisms engaged by retinal electrical stimulation. Invest Ophthalmol Vis Sci. 2006;47:2606–12.

Mccarthy C, Feng D, Barnes N. Augmenting intensity to enhance scene structure in prosthetic vision. In: 2013 IEEE international conference on multimedia and expo workshops (ICMEW), 15–19 July 2013. p. 1–6.

Meister M, Berry MJ 2nd. The neural code of the retina. Neuron. 1999;22:435–50.

Monge M, Raj M, Nazari MH, Chang HC, Zhao Y, Weiland JD, Humayun MS, Tai YC, Emami A. A fully intraocular high-density self-calibrating epiretinal prosthesis. IEEE Trans Biomed Circuits Syst. 2013;7:747–60.

Nanduri D, Fine I, Greenberg RJ, Horsager A, Boynton GM, Weiland JD. Predicting the percepts of electrical stimulation in retinal prosthesis subjects. In: Computational and systems neuroscience meeting, 2011.

Nanduri D, Fine I, Horsager A, Boynton GM, Humayun MS, Greenberg RJ, Weiland JD. Frequency and amplitude modulation have different effects on the percepts elicited by retinal stimulation. Invest Ophthalmol Vis Sci. 2012;53:205–14.

Nasiatka PJ, Mcintosh BP, Stiles NRB, Hauer MC, Weiland JD, Humayun MS, Tanguay AR Jr. An intraocular camera for provision of natural foveation in retinal prostheses. In: Neural interfaces conference, Long Beach, CA, 2010.

Olmedo-Payá A, Martínez-Álvarez A, Cuenca-Asensi S, Ferrández JM, Fernández E. Modeling the role of fixational eye movements in real-world scenes. Neurocomputing. 2015;151(Part 1):78–84.

Ortmanns M, Unger N, Rocke A, Gehrke M, Tietdke HJ. A 0.1 mm/Sup 2/, digitally programmable nerve stimulation pad cell with high-voltage capability for a retinal implant. In: 2006 IEEE international solid state circuits conference – digest of technical papers, 6–9 Feb 2006, 2006. p. 89–98.

Palanker D, Vankov A, Huie P, Baccus S. Design of a high-resolution optoelectronic retinal prosthesis. J Neural Eng. 2005;2:S105–20.

Pradeep V, Medioni G, Weiland J. Visual loop closing using multi-resolution SIFT grids in metric-topological SLAM. In: IEEE conference on computer vision and pattern recognition, 2009 (CVPR 2009), 20–25 June 2009, 2009. p. 1438–45.

Rose TL, Robblee LS. Electrical stimulation with Pt electrodes. VIII. Electrochemically safe charge injection limits with 0.2 ms pulses. IEEE Trans Biomed Eng. 1990;37:1118–20.

Schuettler M, Ordonez JS, Silva Santisteban T, Schatz A, Wilde J, Stieglitz T. Fabrication and test of a hermetic miniature implant package with 360 electrical feedthroughs. Conf Proc IEEE Eng Med Biol Soc. 2010;2010:1585–8.

Sekirnjak C, Hottowy P, Sher A, Dabrowski W, Litke AM, Chichilnisky EJ. Electrical stimulation of mammalian retinal ganglion cells with multielectrode arrays. J Neurophysiol. 2006;95:3311–27.

Sharma A, Rieth L, Tathireddy P, Harrison R, Oppermann H, Klein M, Topper M, Jung E, Normann R, Clark G, Solzbacher F. Evaluation of the packaging and encapsulation reliability in fully integrated, fully wireless 100 channel Utah Slant Electrode Array (USEA): implications for long term functionality. Sens Actuators A Phys. 2012;188:167–72.

Shire DB, Ellersick W, Kelly SK, Doyle P, Priplata A, Drohan W, Mendoza O, Gingerich M, Mckee B, Wyatt JL, Rizzo JF. ASIC design and data communications for the Boston retinal prosthesis. Conf Proc IEEE Eng Med Biol Soc. 2012;2012:292–5.

Stingl K, Bartz-Schmidt KU, Besch D, Braun A, Bruckmann A, Gekeler F, Greppmaier U, Hipp S, Hortdorfer G, Kernstock C, Koitschev A, Kusnyerik A, Sachs H, Schatz A, Stingl KT, Peters T, Wilhelm B, Zrenner E. Artificial vision with wirelessly powered subretinal electronic implant alpha-IMS. Proc Biol Sci. 2013;280:20130077.

Stingl K, Bartz-Schmidt KU, Besch D, Chee CK, Cottriall CL, Gekeler F, Groppe M, Jackson TL, Maclaren RE, Koitschev A, Kusnyerik A, Neffendorf J, Nemeth J, Naeem MA, Peters T, Ramsden JD, Sachs H, Simpson A, Singh MS, Wilhelm B, Wong D, Zrenner E. Subretinal visual implant alpha IMS—clinical trial interim report. Vis Res. 2015;111:149–60.

Suaning GJ, Lavoie P, Forrester J, Armitage T, Lovell NH. Microelectronic retinal prosthesis: III. A new method for fabrication of high-density hermetic feedthroughs. Conf Proc IEEE Eng Med Biol Soc. 2006;1:1638–41.

Suesserman MF, Spelman FA, Rubinstein JT. In vitro measurement and characterization of current density profiles produced by nonrecessed, simple recessed, and radially varying recessed stimulating electrodes. IEEE Trans Biomed Eng. 1991;38:401–8.

Van Rullen R, Thorpe SJ. Rate coding versus temporal order coding: what the retinal ganglion cells tell the visual cortex. Neural Comput. 2001;13:1255–83.

Vanhoestenberghe A, Donaldson N. Corrosion of silicon integrated circuits and lifetime predictions in implantable electronic devices. J Neural Eng. 2013;10:031002.

Wang G, Liu W, Sivaprakasam M, Zhou M, Weiland JD, Humayun MS. A dual band wireless power and data telemetry for retinal prosthesis. Conf Proc IEEE Eng Med Biol Soc. 2006;1:4392–5.

Weiland JD, Humayun MS. Retinal prosthesis. IEEE Trans Biomed Eng. 2014;61:1412–24.

Weiland JD, Anderson DJ, Humayun MS. In vitro electrical properties for iridium oxide versus titanium nitride stimulating electrodes. IEEE Trans Biomed Eng. 2002;49:1574–9.

Weiland JD, Kimock FM, Yehoda JE, Gill E, McIntosh BP, Nasiatka PJ, Tanguay AR. Chip-scale packaging for bioelectronic implants. In: 2013 6th international IEEE/EMBS conference on neural engineering (NER), 6–8 Nov 2013, 2013. p. 931–6.

Weitz AC, Behrend MR, Lee NS, Klein RL, Chiodo VA, Hauswirth WW, Humayun MS, Weiland JD, Chow RH. Imaging the response of the retina to electrical stimulation with genetically encoded calcium indicators. J Neurophysiol. 2013;109:1979–88.

Weitz AC, Behrend MR, Ahuja AK, Christopher P, Wei J, Wuyyuru V, Patel U, Greenberg RJ, Humayun MS, Chow RH, Weiland JD. Interphase gap as a means to reduce electrical stimulation thresholds for epiretinal prostheses. J Neural Eng. 2014;11:–016007.

Wilke RG, Moghadam GK, Lovell NH, Suaning GJ, Dokos S. Electric crosstalk impairs spatial resolution of multi-electrode arrays in retinal implants. J Neural Eng. 2011;8:046016.

Xiao X, Wang J, Liu C, Carlisle JA, Mech B, Greenberg R, Guven D, Freda R, Humayun MS, Weiland J, Auciello O. In vitro and in vivo evaluation of ultrananocrystalline diamond for coating of implantable retinal microchips. J Biomed Mater Res B Appl Biomater. 2006;77:273–81.

Yue L, Weiland JD, Roska B, Humayun MS. Retinal stimulation strategies to restore vision: fundamentals and systems. Prog Retin Eye Res. 2016;53:21–47.

Zhang Y, Rauen SL, Koss M, Calle A, Diniz B, Swenson S, Markland FS, Ufer S, Eckhardt H, Humayun MS, Weiland JD. Wide-field retinal prosthesis with three dimensional, contoured, silicone/polyimide substrates. In: IEEE neural engineering conference, San diego, CA, 2013.

Zhou M, Yuce MR, Liu W. A non-coherent DPSK data receiver with interference cancellation for dual-band transcutaneous telemetries. IEEE J Solid State Circuits. 2008;43:2003–12.

Zhou DD, Dorn JD, Greenberg RJ. The Argus II retinal prosthesis system: an overview. In: IEEE ICME conference, San Jose, CA, 2013.

Chapter 3
Retinal Prostheses: Patient Selection and Screening

Ninel Gregori and Lisa C. Olmos de Koo

Approved Indications for Use

The Argus II Retinal Prosthesis System (Second Sight Medical Products, Inc., Sylmar, CA, USA) is approved for treatment of blindness due to end-stage retinitis pigmentosa (RP) in the United States and any severe outer retinal degeneration in Europe, Saudi Arabia, and Canada. The Argus II system delivers electrical stimulation to residual functioning ganglion cells of degenerated retina which has lost photoreceptors to induce visual perception in patients who meet the following approved criteria: at least 25 years of age, bare light or no light perception in both eyes (if the patient has no residual light perception, evidence of intact inner retinal function must be confirmed as described in Visual Assessment Section below), previous history of useful form vision, pseudophakic or aphakic status, and ability to receive the recommended post-implant clinical follow-up, device fitting, and visual rehabilitation (http://www.secondsight.com/121-the-important-safety-information.html, accessed 12-3-2016). The Argus II prosthesis is intended to be implanted unilaterally, typically in the worse-seeing eye (Ho et al. 2015; da Cruz et al. 2016).

Due to such factors as spatial interaction between electrodes and severity of retinal degeneration, the resolution provided by the present-day retinal prosthesis is limited (Horsager et al. 2011). The artificial vision produced by the Argus II appears as pixelated, shimmering lights, which the patient must learn to interpret as objects. The

N. Gregori, M.D. (✉)
Bascom Palmer Eye Institute, Department of Ophthalmology, University of Miami Miller School of Medicine, Miami, FL, USA
e-mail: ngregori@med.miami.edu

L.C. Olmos de Koo, M.D., M.B.A.
University of Washington Eye Institute, Seattle, WA, USA
e-mail: lolmos@uw.edu

© Springer International Publishing AG 2018
M.S. Humayun, L.C. Olmos de Koo (eds.), *Retinal Prosthesis*, Essentials in Ophthalmology, https://doi.org/10.1007/978-3-319-67260-1_3

system was tested and approved for patients with profoundly limited vision, no better than bare light perception. This level of vision maximizes a chance that the subject will benefit from the prosthetic vision. It has been reported that after implantation, the majority of Argus II patients (93–96%) are able to recognize simple stimuli such as large, high-contrast shapes or large-print letters. More than half (50–60% of patients) also achieve success in more complex tasks, such as detecting direction of a moving bar or following a maze on the floor (Humayun et al. 2012; Stronks and Dagnelie 2014).

The approved baseline vision is bare light perception or worse in both eyes. Based on the results of the clinical trials, a third to a half of Argus II recipients were able to reliably score better than 2.9 logMAR (equivalent to 20/16,000 on the Snellen acuity scale) with the system ON up to 24 months after implantation, and the best result was 1.8 logMAR (equivalent to Snellen 20/1262) (Humayun et al. 2012; da Cruz et al. 2016). The acuity of 2.9 logMAR is the lowest acuity that can be measured with the Berkeley Rudimentary Vision Test (BRVT) Grating Acuity cards that allow quantification of visual acuity in patients unable to read the standard Snellen chart (Bailey et al. 2012). In a prospective trial, approximately 50% of 21 tested subjects with the Argus II device were able to recognize large-print letters (41°) presented on an LCD screen, and four were able to read short words (da Cruz et al. 2013).

By requiring a history of previous useful vision, the presence of a fully developed and functional central visual pathway is likely. A normally functioning visual system is further confirmed by eliciting a history of previous ability to use vision for learning and reading. Congenital or early childhood blindness and profound amblyopia represent contraindications to the Argus II retinal implant.

The patient should be aphakic or pseudophakic to accommodate the implant and allow for adequate visualization of the intraocular components postoperatively. If the patient is phakic, the natural crystalline lens is removed prior to or during the implant procedure by either phacoemulsification or lensectomy approach. If the intraocular lens implant is unstable prior to or during Argus II implantation, the lens implant should be removed during Argus II implantation.

Optimal Ocular Health Considerations

Contraindications to the current Argus II Retinal Prosthesis include ocular diseases or conditions that could affect the integrity of the inner retina or optic nerve required to conduct the signal from the electrodes, such as optic nerve disease, profound amblyopia, trauma, central retinal artery or vein occlusion, or history of retinal detachment. In addition, while not specifically listed as a contraindication, severe strabismus or nystagmus with inability to control eye movements while scanning the environment by head movements should be considered carefully when evaluating the suitability of the Argus II system for a particular patient. The ability to fixate the eye straight ahead helps to align the transmitting and receiving coils and improve the efficiency of the wireless signal transmission. However, many patients with small-angle strabismus and low-amplitude nystagmus have been successfully implanted.

Other contraindications include conditions that could prevent successful implantation. These include extremely thin or scarred conjunctiva that would make covering of the implant difficult; severe ocular surface disease that would cause postoperative dry eye, pain, and conjunctival compromise; axial length outside the required window of 20.5-26.0 mm necessary to accommodate the current prosthesis design; choroidal neovascularization in the area of the intended tack location that could lead to bleeding; posterior staphyloma that would prevent adequate electrode array apposition to the posterior pole, or corneal opacity that would prevent adequate visualization of the retina intraoperatively or postoperatively. A predisposition to eye rubbing can lead to postoperative device exposure and should be addressed preoperatively. Patients with history of significant eye rubbing should not be implanted, due to safety concerns.

Systemic and Mental Health Considerations

Because the implantation surgery can last up to 4 hours, patients with the inability to tolerate general anesthesia cannot undergo implantation. Metallic or active implantable devices in the head, such as cochlear implants, may interfere with device functionality and should be avoided.

Any disease or condition that prevents understanding of the informed consent, fitting of the Argus II system, or postoperative follow-up and rehabilitation is a contraindication. Examples include developmental disability or dementia. Hearing loss is not an absolute contraindication, as long as the patient is able to participate in the fitting and rehabilitation. However, the compatibility of hearing aids with the Argus II glasses should be confirmed prior to surgery. In fact, several Usher syndrome patients have been implanted successfully.

A preoperative psychological evaluation may be recommended based on a physician's assessment and communication with the patient at the screening visit. Currently, there are no specific criteria available for ruling out a poor candidate from psychological standpoint, but it has been observed that patient's personality plays a role in the ability and willingness to undergo an intensive rehabilitation process (Stingl et al. 2013). Additionally, the patient and family must be informed that individuals implanted with an Argus II prosthesis may not undergo electroconvulsive therapy (ECT), which may cause tissue damage or permanent damage to the implant. Thus, anyone with a psychiatric condition requiring treatment with ECT is not a good candidate.

Individuals with central nervous system disease must be made aware of restrictions to magnetic resonance imaging (MRI) parameters deemed safe with the Argus II implant (Weiland et al. 2012). Per the Argus II Product Insert (www.2-sight.com), recipients may undergo MRI only if it is performed using a 1.5 or 3.0 T MRI system. Individuals who may require MRIs with different parameters should consult their physician to discuss the implications for their ability to have scans postoperatively. If suspected, it is also important to rule out organic causes such as stroke or hemorrhage within the central nervous system that may cause a visual field defect and prevent full spectrum of percepts spanning the central 22° provided by the Argus II electrode array.

Finally, the use of the Argus II system during pregnancy and nursing has not been evaluated and should be discussed with females of reproductive age.

Managing Patient Expectations

A critical aspect of patient selection is establishing realistic patient expectations regarding device functionality and expected prosthetic vision. In order to best manage patient expectations, the screening physician should directly ask the patient what he/she hopes to gain with the system. Common answers are seeing a loved one's face, driving a car, or reading a book. However, at the present time, none of these visual tasks are possible. For instance, the pixelated artificial vision may allow the patient to visualize the shape of the person but not the fine features of a person's face. Patients should be informed that they will not be able to read at a normal speed, drive a car, or recognize fine details of an object. In the clinical trial and after device commercialization, patients have been able to visualize large, high-contrast object such as the doors, windows, people, moon, fireworks, and crosswalk lines. Color vision is not currently expected with standard device use, as phosphenes are typically seen as bright or white.

The physician should explain to the patient that the artificial vision generated by the device and the vision the patient had prior to losing sight are quite different. The artificial vision typically consists of pixelated lights, often shimmering, which the patient must learn to interpret as objects that have meaning. This process takes time and patience, and it is analogous to putting the pieces of a puzzle together with some pieces missing. At first, the artificial phosphenes the patient sees may be difficult to interpret, but with continued practice, the brain learns to form mental images. The patient must continue practicing every day, and thus blind rehabilitation is an integral part of the process.

Another critical aspect to convey is that any residual vision could decline in the implanted eye. It is helpful to ask the patient whether he or she has any useful residual vision. Can the patient locate objects at home, such as windows and lamps? Can the patient follow the lines of a crosswalk or detect obstacles when walking? Can the patient use his or her vision to participate in sports or hobbies? If the answer to any of these questions is "yes," the patient may not derive useful benefit from the system.

Reviewing these factors, particularly with patients who have high expectations from the Argus II, may be challenging and time-consuming for the screening physician, but it is critical to establish realistic expectations so that patients who will not benefit are spared from the significant burden of surgery, device cost, and time spent in rehabilitation.

Just as patients seeking a retinal implant may have unrealistic expectations about what they will be able to see after implantation, they may also have unrealistic expectations about the amount of effort and work they will need to put forth in order for the device to benefit them. Prospective patients should understand that diligence and a firm commitment to learning to use the device are essential in order to obtain the best results. The patient must be informed that the Argus II Retinal Prosthesis System is not meant to replace the other visual aids a patient may already be using, such as a cane or a dog, but is another useful aid to help their mobility and independence.

The degree of visual impairment in outer retinal degenerations is highly variable, and only patients with profound visual loss are currently good candidates for the Argus II. Clinical trials have shown that there appears to be some degree of variability in patients' acceptance of the implanted device (da Cruz et al. 2013). Quality of life studies have shown that patients whose blindness has negatively impacted such quality of life aspects as injury avoidance, copying with the demands of life, and fulfilling life roles reported significant long-term, durable (over 36 months) improvement after Argus II implantation (Duncan et al. 2016).

Conducting Patient Screening

Upon confirmation that the patient meets the criteria for on-label use (age at least 25 years old, diagnosis of severe retinitis pigmentosa (United States) or an outer retinal degeneration, and history of previous useful vision), the screening process is initiated. Screening typically involves a standardized survey, patient interview, and complete eye exam, including biometry, optional B-scan ultrasonography, and macular OCT as described below. The following steps have been used by screening physicians. The screening process may be discontinued at any point if the patient is deemed ineligible.

Visual Function Assessment

Perform a *visual function assessment* to confirm that the patient has bare light or no light perception in both eyes. If there is no light perception, photoflash testing or electrically evoked response may be used to confirm the function of the inner retina and optic nerve. Patients with profound amblyopia may not benefit due to a lack of development of the visual cortex. The visual function assessment, though it may sound simple, is in fact one of the most critical screening steps, and care should be taken to ensure accurate results, using both objective and subjective assessments. As such, the physician may consider verifying the results if they were obtained by a technician or other designees.

To confirm that the patient has vision no better than bare light perception, standard clinical measures of visual function (ETDRS or Snellen chart, count fingers/hand motion/light perception) *and/or* the Berkeley Rudimentary Vision Test (BVRT) can be used (Section "Standard Clinical Measures of Visual Function and/or

Berkeley Rudimentary Vision Test (BRVT)" below). The results of either of these tests may also establish that the patient has a functioning visual system (i.e., he/she can detect bright light). If light perception is still ambiguous, one can use the photoflash test (see "Photoflash Test" below) or electrically evoked responses (see "Confirming Inner Retina Functionality by Electrically Evoked Response (EER)" below) to establish the health of the remaining visual system.

Each eye should be tested separately while the patient looks straight ahead in order to test central acuity. If it is apparent that the patient is using peripheral vision, a further exploration of the extent and usefulness of the peripheral vision is warranted with visual field measurement and/or the residual vision interview (see Section "Residual Vision Interview").

Standard Clinical Measures of Visual Function and/or Berkeley Rudimentary Vision Test (BRVT)

The visual assessment described below may be used to verify bare light perception or no light perception vision, but the screening physician should use his or her judgment based on the clinical evaluation of the patient as to whether all steps are indicated or applicable. As part of the standard clinical measures of visual function, one may choose to test whether the patient is able to read any rows on a standard *vision chart* at 1 m, *count fingers* at 1 foot, or determine the *direction of hand motion* 1 foot away. If the patient is unable to perform those tasks, light perception should be verified. In a dark room, a bright penlight, muscle light, or indirect ophthalmoscope light is used to shine a focused light directly into patient's eye. The light is moved into and away from the eye several times to verify. If the patient cannot detect any light, a photoflash test (Section "Photoflash Test") may be necessary to establish intact visual system function.

The BRVT is a visual function test for vision worse than that measured by the ETDRS chart (Bailey et al. 2012). While it was not used in the Argus II clinical trial, it may be useful for evaluating implant candidates in a post-market setting instead of or in addition to a standard clinical evaluation of low vision (i.e., counting fingers, hand motion, light perception).

Regardless of the method used to assess residual visual function, if the results are ambiguous, as they may be in this very low vision group, who have adapted other senses to compensate for their lack of vision, a careful discussion with the patient to assess their residual functional vision will help the screening physician to make the final decision.

Berkeley Rudimentary Vision Test (BRVT) Procedure

The test involves 16 steps, which are followed separately for each eye while patching the non-tested eye. Room light is kept bright except for step 1 (testing light perception). Steps 2–16 utilize various optotypes of increasing difficulty to document the maximum visual acuity of the patient. The second step tests whether the patient is able to detect a white versus a black card. In the third step, the patient is asked to identify whether the top or the bottom half of the page is white versus black. In the fourth step, the patient determines which quarter of the page is white (top left, top right, bottom right, or bottom left). In steps 5–16, the patient is asked to determine the orientation of bars in the Grating Acuity cards (vertical or horizontal bars) and the direction of letter E in the Tumbling E cards (up, down, right, or left). The minimal acuity is quantified with the Grating 200 M cards (equivalent to 2.9 logMAR) shown at a distance of 25 cm from the patient. The maximal acuity is quantified with the Tumbling E 25M cards (1.4 logMAR) held 1 m from the patient.

For step 1, light perception is tested in a dark room using a bright penlight or similar small, focused light. The patient is asked when (s)he sees a light. For each trial, the penlight is moved until it is shining directly into the tested eye. If the patient reports seeing a light quickly, within seconds after the light is shone in the eye, that trial is recorded as correct. Repeat this test six times, with different amounts of time (from 2 to 10 s) in between each trial. If the patient reports seeing a light at any time when no light is shone into the eye, the trial is recorded as incorrect.

For all other steps, the room lights should be on; the specified optotype is presented at a random orientation six times for each eye. For each trial, the patient's response is recorded as correct or incorrect. Second sight testing kit contains instructions on the criteria that are followed to determine whether to advance to the next step. The visual acuity for the tested eye is equal to the vision corresponding to the step where the screening was stopped.

If the patient is unable to reliably detect a penlight, a photoflash test (Section "Photoflash Test" below) may be done to establish intact visual system function. If he or she is able to advance through the first few BRVT steps only, the patient may be eligible based on the results of the residual vision questionnaire and functional assessment (Sections "Residual Vision Interview" and "Residual Vision Functional Assessment" below). If the patient is able to advance through the last few steps involving Tumbling E cards, he or she likely has residual vision that is better than bare light perception. If the results of the visual function tests are not clear, extra effort to investigate patient's vision with the residual vision interview and residual vision functional assessment (Sections "Residual Vision Interview" and "Residual Vision Functional Assessment" below) would be warranted.

Photoflash Test

The patient's eyes should be dilated and dark adapted for 20 min, and the flash test should be performed in a dark room. The fellow eye is patched during testing. To reduce waiting time, one may wish to try it first without dark adaption of the eyes and only use dark adaptation if the patient is clearly unable to see the flash.

The patient is instructed that for each trial, he or she will hear the flash go off four times, but the flash will only be illuminated one of the four times. The patient is asked to announce in which interval he/she saw the light. The photoflash kit contains a suggested testing sequence indicating in which interval the flash should be applied in front of the subject. For some patients, one may need to wait for up to a minute between each interval and trial, so the patient does not confuse new flashes with previous flashes. For each trial, the interval where patient announced he/she sees light is recorded. A correct response is where the subject answers positively to the interval in which the flash actually occurred. An incorrect response is where the subject answers positively to an interval in which the flash did not occur. One can stop the test if/when the subject reaches nine correct answers. If the patient scores correctly on nine or more trials, the vision is recorded as bare light perception. If the patient scores correctly on less than nine trials, the vision is recorded as no light perception.

Confirming Inner Retina Functionality by Electrically Evoked Response (EER)

In the rare occasion that the patient is unable to detect any flashes in the photoflash test, one needs to determine whether or not residual bipolar and ganglion cells are capable of properly forwarding electrical signals from the electrodes (Stingl et al. 2013). Retinal excitability can be measured by means of electrically evoked response (EER) via a corneal electrode (Stingl et al. 2013). This test is only performed during screening of the eye intended for implantation and only if the patient has no light detection on the photoflash test.

The necessary equipment includes Digitimer constant current stimulator (Model number DS7A), Second Sight EER electrode (Catalog Number 130160-001), 1 cm diameter Grass electrode, Goniosol, and eye patches.

EER Procedure

- The cornea is anesthetized with topical anesthesia, and the EER disposable electrode is placed on the eye with Goniosol. The lead wire is taped to the cheek.
- The area behind the ear on the tested side of the head is cleaned with alcohol. A 1 cm diameter Grass electrode is placed behind the ear with electrode gel, and the lead wire is taped to the neck. This electrode is used as the reference.
- The non-tested eye is patched.
- Testing is commenced with the stimulation amplitude set at 1 mA with a pulse width of 1 ms. Current is passed between the electrode and the common electrode in a single pulse. The subject is asked if they perceived any light at the moment of stimulation. The stimulation pulse is repeated eight times, and the number of positive responses is recorded. If the subject does not perceive light on at least five of the presentations, the stimulus amplitude is increased in steps of 1 mA, up to a maximum of 8 mA. If at 8 mA the subject fails to perceive light on at least five of the presentations, the pulse width is increased to 2 milliseconds (ms) and the test is repeated, starting at a stimulus amplitude of 1 mA and increasing in 1 mA steps to 8 mA if necessary.

- If the subject does not perceive light on at least five out of eight presentations of the 8 mA 2 ms pulse, he/she is classified as having insufficient optic nerve function in that eye and is excluded from implantation.

Residual Vision Interview

These and similar questions can be used to gain an understanding of whether the patient believes he or she has useful residual vision. This is critical since the residual vision may decline after implantation in that eye. The following questions have been used by Argus II surgeons for screening purposes:

- Does the patient report having any residual vision?
- If yes, what does he/she report being able to do with it? Can he/she use it for visual tasks in the real world?
- Can he/she use residual vision for orientation tasks, such as determining the location of windows, ceiling lights, or lamps?
- Can he/she use residual vision for mobility tasks such as following the lines of a crosswalk or detecting obstacles?
- Can he/she use residual vision to do sports or hobbies?
- Would he or she be willing to accept the potential risk of experiencing a decline in or loss of the residual vision in the implanted eye?

Residual Vision Functional Assessment

The following questions can be used to gain an understanding of whether the patient is able to use his or her residual vision to perform basic visual tasks and, if so, whether the vision is central or peripheral:

- The room light is brightly lit, and the patient is asked if he/she can visually determine anything about the environment—light locations, people moving, etc.
- If the patient can see features of the environment, he/she is asked to describe where (in the visual field) he/she has vision.
- The patient should be observed to determine whether he or she has a preferred retinal locus: consistently not looking straight ahead while trying to use residual vision or keeping the head to one side may be a sign of residual vision.

Comprehensive Eye Exam

Perform a *comprehensive eye exam (both eyes)*, assessing whether or not any contraindications are present. Lids should be evaluated for any abnormalities including significant blepharitis, which should be treated to minimize risk of postoperative infection. The conjunctiva is evaluated to rule out extreme thinning or scarring. Gentle movement of the conjunctiva with a cotton swab after installation of an anesthetic drop is helpful. The cornea is inspected to rule out significant opacity that prevents visualization of the retina. The lens status is evaluated, and intraocular lens subluxation or instability should be documented to help the decision of whether it should be removed. If a crystalline lens is present, the patient should be informed of the necessity to remove it during or before the Argus II implantation. The posterior pole is evaluated to rule out staphyloma, retinal detachment, or any other pathology. The status of the optic nerve should be documented, and any disease such as glaucoma that may prevent the conduction of the signal to the brain should be ruled out.

Medical History

Review the *medical history*. The surgeon must ensure that the patient meets all of the eligibility criteria contained in the product label, there are no contraindications to device placement, the patient's level of residual vision contributes to a favorable risk/benefit profile, and the patient's motivations, expectations, cognitive and communication skills, and physical abilities are likely to contribute to receiving benefit from the device. Medical history is reviewed for contraindications such as metallic or active implantable device (e.g., cochlear implant) in the head and ocular conditions that would prevent implantation, healing, visualization, or performance of the Argus II implant.

Motivation and Expectations

Question the patient regarding *motivation and expectations*. Counsel the patient about the time and the effort required to undergo vision rehabilitation. Patients who live very far from the clinic who do not have transportation or who do not understand the requirement for follow-up visits may be more likely to be dissatisfied with the Argus II system after implant. It is important to gain an understanding of the patient's availability for and commitment to the requirements for fitting and rehabilitation.

It is possible that patients with greater independence and those who have shown high motivation to seek out and learn from blind rehabilitation may be more satisfied with vision from the Argus II. Conversely, those with very high expectations of the system are more likely to be disappointed. The physician should utilize his/her judgment to determine this.

The patient should be informed that that there will be up to five visits to the clinic in the first month, with roughly one visit a week with a rehabilitation therapist (in the clinic or at the patient's home) for the following 1.5–2 months. Long-term visits (one per year or more) will also be required for medical follow-up and re-fitting.

The patient should understand that hard work is part of the process and a firm commitment to it is required to get the best result.

Testing the Glasses and Video Processing Unit

The patient should be allowed to try on the Argus II glasses and feel the wearable components of the external device. In some rare cases, the style or fit of the glasses could be a source of patient dissatisfaction post-implant if s(he) was not introduced to them prior to surgery. The patient should be allowed to touch and wear the glasses and VPU.

Applanation A-Scan Ultrasonography with Biometry

Perform *applanation A-scan ultrasonography with biometry* to measure the axial length. An applanation probe at ≥10 MHz (preferred over noncontact optical devices) is performed five times along the optical axis, and the average of five measurements is calculated for each eye. Measurements may be difficult due to a poor ability to fixate and must be done carefully. If the length is <20.5 mm or >26.0 mm, the patient is not eligible for the current implant. The axial length sets several important surgical implantation landmarks; thus, accuracy is critical.

Diagnostic B-Scan Ultrasonography Imaging

Perform optional *diagnostic B-scan ultrasonography imaging* to rule out a staphyloma. The electrode array may not make a good contact with the retinal surface in cases of staphyloma, leading to higher electrical thresholds and poor device functionality. If the patient is enrolled in the post-approval study conducted for 5 years after Argus II implantation to collect device safety, functional vision, visual acuity, and device performance data, the thickness of the posterior ocular coats is measured three times and the average is taken.

Spectral-Domain Macular Optical Coherence Tomography

Perform *spectral-domain macular optical coherence tomography* (OCT) to evaluate the retinal layers and rule out any significant protrusions or depressions in the macula, which could affect how well the Argus II array fits against the retina. Such conditions as a staphyloma, macular scarring with distorted inner retinal contour, and significant epiretinal membranes must be noted. Close contact between the electrodes and the inner retina is essential for the optimal electric stimulation of the ganglion cells.

Fundus and External Reflex Photography

The physician may also consider an optional color 50° field *fundus photography as well as external reflex photography* to document the natural position of the eye and any strabismus present.

Risks and Probable Benefit

Review the *risks and probable benefit* again with the patient. If the patient is eligible and interested, follow your institutional procedures for consenting, scheduling, and ordering the device. Humanitarian Use Device (HUD) IRB consent is required for implantation in the United States.

Nonqualifiers

Patients with RP or other outer retinal degenerations who do not qualify for the device fall into two basic categories: those who are unlikely to become candidates in the future due to anatomic considerations or other pathology and those who do not qualify because of useful residual vision. This second group may take comfort in the knowledge that future device improvements may make it helpful to those with better vision. Furthermore, should their vision continue to decline, the Argus II represents a "safety net" against the complete blindness encountered by some of these patients. Nevertheless, even those who do not qualify for this particular device because of anatomic considerations or other pathology should be encouraged that ophthalmic research continues to yield promising future therapies.

Conclusion

In summary, screening potential candidates for Argus II implantation involves careful patient evaluation, education, and counseling in this unique, profoundly blind population. A trained technician conducts a visual assessment with standard and specialized tests. The dimensions of the eye are measured to determine the likelihood for successful implantation and healing. Patient history, psychological, and general health factors are carefully evaluated. A detailed ophthalmic exam is performed. The implanting surgeon must be responsible for ensuring that all factors will contribute to device functionality and acceptance by the patient. Proper patient screening and counseling are vital parts of success in Argus II implantation.

Compliance with Ethical Requirements Ninel Z. Gregori and Lisa C. Olmos de Koo declare that they have no relevant conflicts of interest. No human or animal studies were carried out by the authors for this article.

References

Bailey IL, Jackson AJ, Minto H, Greer RB, Chu MA. The Berkeley rudimentary vision test. Optom Vis Sci. 2012;89(9):1257–64.

da Cruz L, Coley BF, Dorn J, Merlini F, Filley E, Christopher P, Chen FK, Wuyyuru V, Sahel J, Stanga P, Humayun M, Greenberg RJ, Dagnelie G, Argus IISG. The Argus II epiretinal prosthesis system allows letter and word reading and long-term function in patients with profound vision loss. Br J Ophthalmol. 2013;97(5):632–6.

da Cruz L, Dorn JD, Humayun MS, Dagnelie G, Handa J, Barale PO, Sahel JA, Stanga PE, Hafezi F, Safran AB, Salzmann J, Santos A, Birch D, Spencer R, Cideciyan AV, de Juan E, Duncan JL, Eliott D, Fawzi A, Olmos de Koo LC, Ho AC, Brown G, Haller J, Regillo C, Del Priore LV, Arditi A, Greenberg RJ, Argus IISG. Five-year safety and performance results from the Argus II retinal prosthesis system clinical trial. Ophthalmology. 2016;123(10):2248–54.

Duncan JL, Richards TP, Arditi A, da Cruz L, Dagnelie G, Dorn JD, Ho AC, Olmos de Koo LC, Barale PO, Stanga PE, Thumann G, Wang Y, Greenberg RJ. Improvements in vision-related quality of life in blind patients implanted with the Argus II Epiretinal Prosthesis. Clin Exp Optom. 2016;100(2):144–50.

Ho AC, Humayun MS, Dorn JD, da Cruz L, Dagnelie G, Handa J, Barale PO, Sahel JA, Stanga PE, Hafezi F, Safran AB, Salzmann J, Santos A, Birch D, Spencer R, Cideciyan AV, de Juan E, Duncan JL, Eliott D, Fawzi A, Olmos de Koo LC, Brown GC, Haller JA, Regillo CD, Del Priore LV, Arditi A, Geruschat DR, Greenberg RJ, Argus IISG. Long-term results from an epiretinal prosthesis to restore sight to the blind. Ophthalmology. 2015;122(8):1547–54.

Horsager A, Boynton GM, Greenberg RJ, Fine I. Temporal interactions during paired-electrode stimulation in two retinal prosthesis subjects. Invest Ophthalmol Vis Sci. 2011;52(1):549–57.

Humayun MS, Dorn JD, da Cruz L, Dagnelie G, Sahel JA, Stanga PE, Cideciyan AV, Duncan JL, Eliott D, Filley E, Ho AC, Santos A, Safran AB, Arditi A, Del Priore LV, Greenberg RJ, Argus IISG. Interim results from the international trial of Second Sight's visual prosthesis. Ophthalmology. 2012;119(4):779–88.

Stingl K, Bach M, Bartz-Schmidt KU, Braun A, Bruckmann A, Gekeler F, Greppmaier U, Hortdorfer G, Kusnyerik A, Peters T, Wilhelm B, Wilke R, Zrenner E. Safety and efficacy of subretinal visual implants in humans: methodological aspects. Clin Exp Optom. 2013;96(1):4–13.

Stronks HC, Dagnelie G. The functional performance of the Argus II retinal prosthesis. Expert Rev Med Devices. 2014;11(1):23–30.

Weiland JD, Faraji B, Greenberg RJ, Humayun MS, Shellock FG. Assessment of MRI issues for the Argus II retinal prosthesis. Magn Reson Imaging. 2012;30(3):382–9.

Chapter 4
Retinal Prostheses: Surgical Techniques and Postoperative Management

Stanislao Rizzo and Laura Cinelli

Argus® II Retinal Prosthesis (Implant)

The Argus® II retinal prosthesis is a medical device surgically implanted in and on the eye. The implant's part located outside of the eye is composed of a scleral band (equivalent to a 240 band used in scleral buckling procedures) on which are encased an implant coil and an electronic case connected to each other.

The implant coil is a receiving and transmitting antenna (made of a gold wire) that communicates wirelessly, via radio frequency, with an external coil mounted on the Argus® II glasses. The electronic case (a group of application-specific integrated circuits) receives data from the implant coil, processes them, and generates the electrical stimulation output that, through the electrode array, reaches the retina.

The implant's part located inside of the eye is composed of a polymer cable (containing the wire conductors) connected, on its proximal end, to the case and, with its distal end, to the array (made of 60 platinum electrodes, 200 μm diameter each, with a silicone covering on the retinal side for tissue protection) (Fig. 4.1).

Fasteners and Grabbing Tools

The Argus® II implant design has been developed for an easy handling and surgical placement.

To anchor the implant to the sclera, three suture tabs are provided: two on the electronic case and one on the implant coil (Fig. 4.2).

S. Rizzo, M.D. (✉) • L. Cinelli, M.D.
Department of Surgery and Translational Medicine, Eye Clinic, University of Florence, Florence, Italy
e-mail: stanislao.rizzo@gmail.com; laucinelli@yahoo.it

© Springer International Publishing AG 2018
M.S. Humayun, L.C. Olmos de Koo (eds.), *Retinal Prosthesis*, Essentials in Ophthalmology, https://doi.org/10.1007/978-3-319-67260-1_4

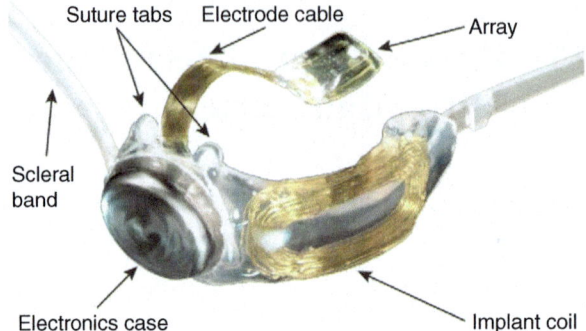

Fig. 4.1 Argus® II implant with its components: receiving implant coil, electronic case, electrode cable, 60-electrode array (image courtesy of Second Sight Medical Products)

Fig. 4.2 Argus® II suture tabs for implant anchorage onto the sclera (image courtesy of Second Sight Medical Products)

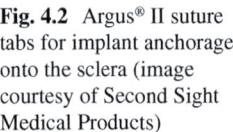

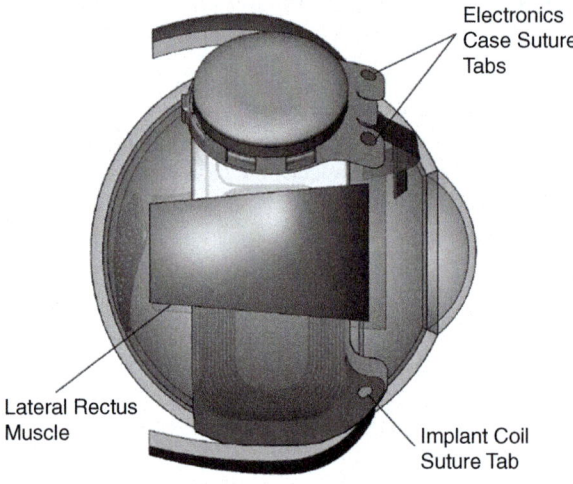

To safely grab the array during insertion maneuvers into the vitreous cavity and its positioning over the macular region, a "handle" on the distal end of the array is provided.

To fix the electrode array over the fovea with the retinal tack specifically created by Second Sight Medical Products, a tack hole on the proximal end of the array is provided (Fig. 4.3).

Equipment and Supplies for Implantation

In order to perform the Argus® II epiretinal implant surgery, the surgeon should use both standard vitreoretinal tools and specifically designed surgical instruments. A series of tools has been carefully selected to allow the clinician to grab and easily

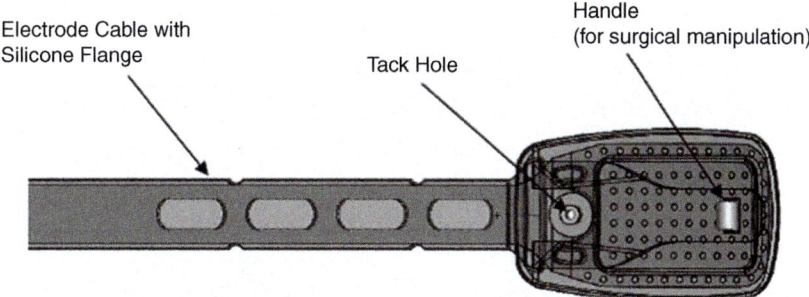

Electrode Cable with
Silicone Flange

Tack Hole

Handle
(for surgical manipulation)

Fig. 4.3 Argus® II handle for surgical manipulation and tack hole for retinal tack insertion (image courtesy of Second Sight Medical Products)

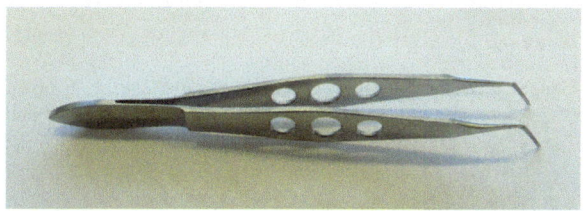

Fig. 4.4 Silicone-tipped forceps (to safely manipulate the implant)

manipulate the implant during the extraocular placement and the intraocular positioning, such as the silicone-tipped forceps (Fig. 4.4) and the 20-gauge end-gripping forceps (Fig. 4.5a and b).

Among the surgical tools created specifically by Second Sight Medical Products for this type of surgery, we find retinal tack forceps 19 gauge (Fig. 4.6a and b) used to catch and insert the tack into the vitreous cavity and retinal tack used to fix the array onto the retina. The tack has a spring on it to keep the array in contact with the retina (Fig. 4.7).

Moreover, you will also need external equipment, provided by Second Sight Medical Products, necessary to test the functionality of the system before, during, and after the implant procedures.

Below you will find a full list of equipment, supplies, and tools that are required to implant the Argus® II device.

Argus® II Implant

Containing:

- One Argus® II implant (sterile)
- Two Argus® II retinal tacks (sterile)

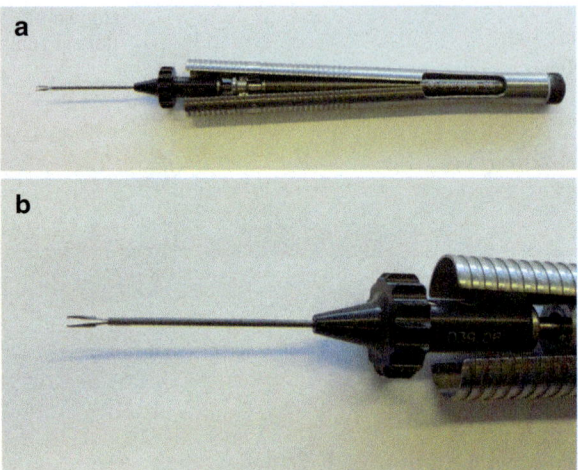

Fig. 4.5 (**a**) 20-Gauge Eckardt end-gripping forceps (to grab the array "handle" during its insertion through the 5.2 sclerotomy and its fixing on the retina. (**b**) Tip of 20-gauge Eckardt end-gripping forceps

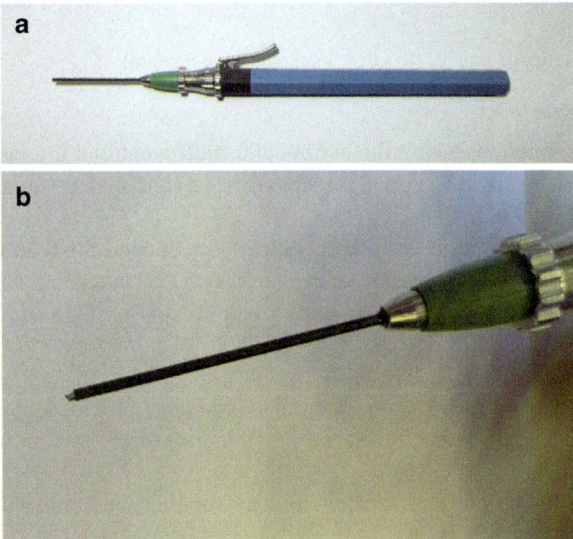

Fig. 4.6 (**a**) 19-Gauge retinal tack forceps (to grab and insert the tack into the vitreous cavity). (**b**) Tip of 19-gauge retinal tack forceps

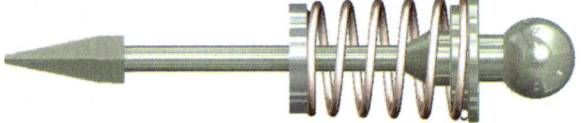

Fig. 4.7 Retinal tack (to fix the array onto the retina)

Argus® II External Devices

Argus® II operating room coil (OR coil)
- Argus® II video-processing unit (VPU)
- Argus® II communication adapter (CA)
- Argus® II clinician fitting system (CFS)
- Cables and accessories:
  - VPU battery
  - Argus® II CA-VPU cable
  - Argus® II CFS-CA cable

Standard Vitreoretinal Surgical Equipment

- Vitrector
- Operating microscope (with inverter)
- Panoramic view system
- Vitrectomy lens(es)
- Bipolar electrosurgical equipment

Surgical Instruments

Gripping

- Silicone-tipped forceps
- End-gripping forceps, 20 gauge
- Retinal tack forceps, 19 gauge
- Fixation forceps
- Suturing forceps
- Tying forceps
- Barraquer's needle holder
- Utility or dressing forceps, serrated jaws
- Utility forceps, smooth jaws
- Watzke sleeve spreading forceps
- Scleral plug forceps

Cutting

- 20-Gauge myringotomy knife
- 5.2 angled bevel up knife
- 15° single edge knife
- Westcott blunt scissors

Others

- Calipers (millimeter increments or smaller)
- Soft-tipped cannula
- Lid speculum
- (2) Muscle hooks, one plain, one with eyelet
- Vitreous cutter
- 25-gauge straight endoillumination probe
- 25-gauge infusion cannula
- 25-gauge chandelier
- 25-gauge trocar, entry system valved

Surgical Supplies

- Silicone sleeves (Labtician Ophthalmics TM, Oval Sleeve, Style #3083)
- 7-0 Vicryl sutures braided with spatula needle or equivalent absorbable sutures to close sclerotomies
- 5-0 Mersilene sutures braided with spatula needle or equivalent nonabsorbable sutures to fix episcleral band and tab holes onto the sclera
- 2-0 Silk sutures or equivalent to pass around muscles
- 8-0 Vicryl sutures or equivalent to close Tenon's capsule and conjunctiva
- 10-0 Ethilon monofil nonabsorbable sutures to close corneal tunnel
- Processed pericardium or equivalent (approximately 400 μm thick)
- Sterile balanced salt solution
- Sterile sleeves/sterile camera drapes
- Spare tack for the electrode array
- Sterile powder-free and latex-free gloves or sterile silicone phaco test chamber
- General vitreoretinal surgical items

Surgical Technique for Argus® II Retinal Prosthesis Implantation

The Argus® II surgical implantation is performed under general anesthesia. The average duration of surgery is about 3 h. Surgery can be divided into five phases (Second Sight Medical Products, Inc. 2013):

1. Preparation
2. Extraocular placement
3. Intraocular placement
4. Closure
5. Intraoperative implant testing procedure

Phase 1: Preparation

The first step for a successful outcome of the surgery is to avoid infection by adhering to scrupulous sterile technique and carefully preparing the eye region at the beginning of the operation. Extra attention should be paid to eyelashes and removal of any debris. Adhere to sterile technique throughout the procedure by limiting the number of personnel in the operating room, limiting the flow of personnel in and out of the room, and requiring all personnel to wear masks that cover the nose and mouth. Administer 8 mg of dexamethasone and 1 g of cefazolin via intravenous infusion to the patient (Table.4.1). Cover the implant, still located inside the tray, with 48 ml of sterile salt solution and antibiotics (add 1 ml of vancomycin and 1 ml of ceftazidime) for 5 min, and then rinse the implant with sterile salt solution before installing it on the eye.

The second step is to remove the lens with phacoemulsification (if the patient is phakic) and leave him aphakic after the procedure. Then close the corneal tunnel with an Ethilon 10-0 suture point. If the patient is pseudophakic, the intraocular lens should be left in place unless it is subluxed or dislocated or has high likelihood of becoming subluxed or dislocated (in which case it should be removed through a limbal incision).

The third step is to perform a 360° limbal conjunctival peritomy as in all ab externo scleral fixation techniques. The Argus® II implant is made specifically for either the left eye or the right eye. In any case, the electronic case must be placed in the supero-temporal quadrant. To avoid dehiscence of the conjunctival wound in correspondence of the implant case, only one radial relaxing incision is made in the inferonasal quadrant or in line with the rectus muscles. The four rectus muscles are isolated with 2-0 silk (Fig. 4.8).

At this point, using silicone-tipped tweezers or forceps, the implant is removed from the tray by sliding the scleral band out from under the two cross bands holding it in the tray and rinsed with sterile salt solution.

Phase 2: Extraocular Placement

Before starting to insert the silicon episcleral band with its incorporated case and coil under the four recti muscles and securing them onto the sclera with sutures, it is important to protect the implant cable and the array from contamination and

Table 4.1 Intra-operative medication

Intraoperative medication	Start of procedure	Intravenous steroid: Dexamethasone 8 mg (or equivalent)
		Intravenous antibiotic: Cefazolin 1 g (or equivalent)
	End of procedure	Intravitreal antibiotics: Vancomycin 1 mg and ceftazidime 2.25 mg (or equivalent)
		Subconjunctival antibiotics: Cefazolin 100 mg and dexamethasone 2 mg (or equivalent)

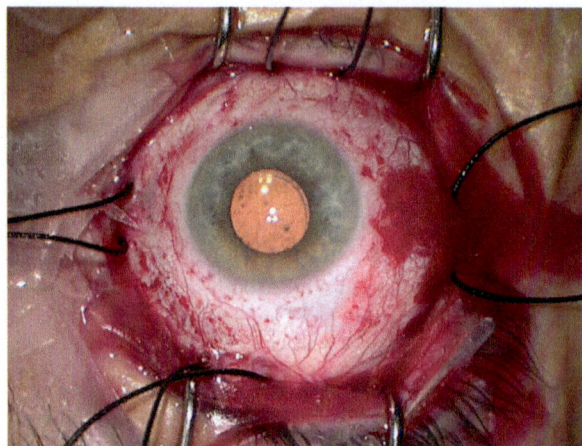

Fig. 4.8 360° limbal conjunctival peritomy and rectus muscle isolation with 2-0 silk suture

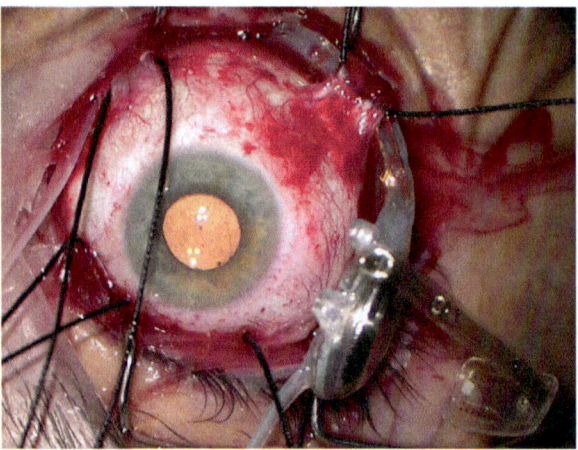

Fig. 4.9 Inserting coil under lateral rectus muscle, placing the electronic case in the supero-temporal quadrant

trauma by covering them with a protecting sleeve (it could be a fingertip cut from a small sterile talc-free glove or a sterile silicone phaco test chamber tip).

At this point, the receiving coil is inserted under the lateral rectus muscle (Fig. 4.9) using fingers or blunt forceps, while the electronic case rests in the supero-temporal quadrant. Then, the inferior part of the scleral band is passed under the inferior and the medial rectus muscles, while the superior portion of the band is passed under the superior rectus muscle. The two ends are then secured with a Watzke sleeve, applied in the superior nasal quadrant (Fig. 4.10).

Next, the encirclement band is sutured with 5-0 Mersilene in the two nasal quadrants, and the electronic parts (transmitting coil and electronic case) are

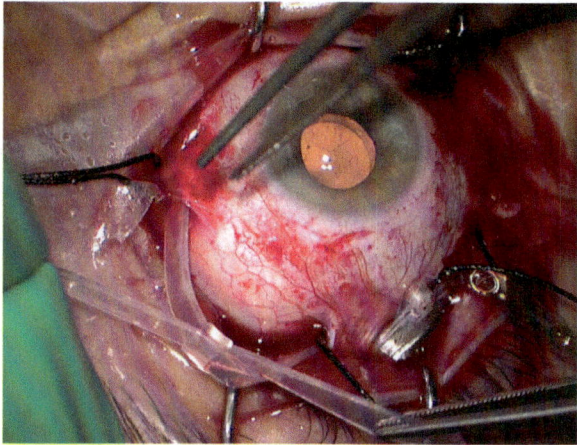

Fig. 4.10   Silicone sleeve is applied in the superior nasal quadrant

temporarily fixed to the sclera with 5-0 Mersilene, using the special tab holes carved on the silicone shell. Suture bites should be taken anterior to posterior, emerging at the intended suture tab hole setback distance provided by special axial length-related tables (Second Sight Medical Products medical product). Before definitively fixing the external implant to the sclera, the surgeon must make sure that the electronic case is centered in the supero-temporal quadrant adjusting the superior/inferior position of the case and that the distances between the suture tab and the limbus are calculated according to the special fitting tables mentioned above, adjusting the anterior/posterior position of the case and coil. It is very important to carefully follow the measurements listed in the table in order to allow enough cable for optimal positioning of the multielectrode array on the retinal surface, above the macula. Once the suture tab hole positions are confirmed, we can permanently tie the sutures by attaching them through the three suture tabs (Figs. 4.11 and 4.12).

Finally, rotate the suture knots so that the cut ends face toward the sclera as much as possible to minimize the risk of conjunctival abrasion.

During this maneuver, the surgeon must be very careful to safeguard every electrical component.

Phase 3: Intraocular Placement

Three scleral ports for the vitrectomy (infusion line inferotemporal, vitrectomy port at 3 and 9 o'clock) are created at 3.5 mm from the limbus, and a complete vitrectomy, with removal of the posterior vitreous, is performed with the aid of a chandelier light. We use the ZEISS Lumera 700 microscope and Constellation vitrectomy

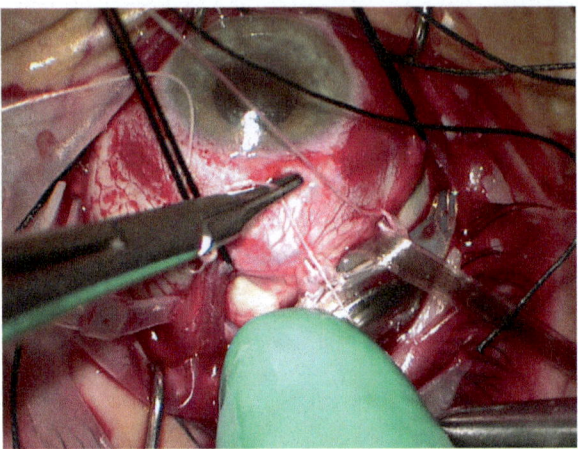

Fig. 4.11 Electronic case anchored with 5-0 Mersilene suture to the sclera in the supero-temporal quadrant using the special tab holes

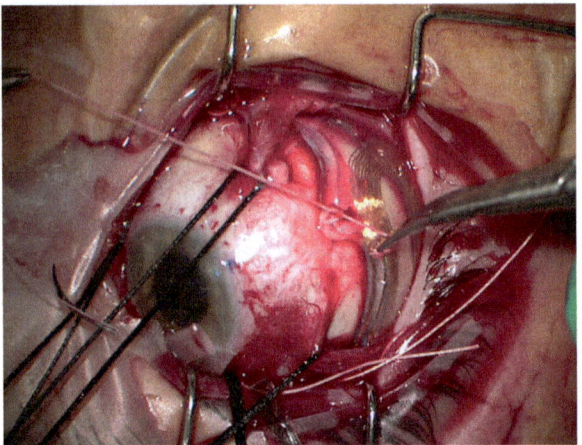

Fig. 4.12 Implant coil anchored to the sclera with 5-0 Mersilene suture in the inferotemporal quadrant using the special tab holes

system (Alcon Fort Worth, USA), using 25-gauge (25 + Series) instruments and valved trocars. The RESIGHT system is used to visualize the retina. After core vitrectomy is performed, triamcinolone acetonide is injected into the vitreous cavity to facilitate visualization of the vitreous and retinal surface. A posterior vitreous detachment is induced, avoiding excessive traction on the retina. The vitreous cortex is usually very adherent in eyes with Retinitis Pigmentosa (especially in young patients) and normally does not detach further than the mid-periphery (Mura and Bamonte 2014).

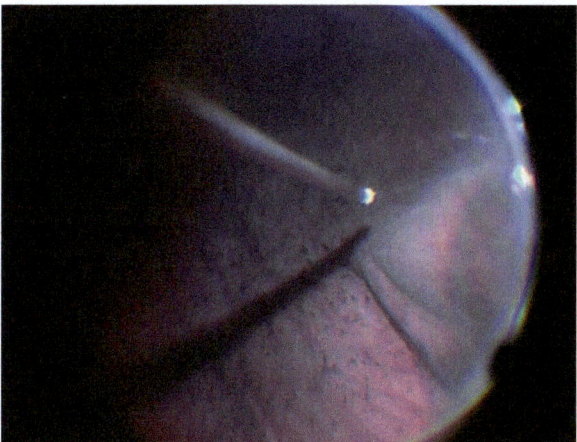

Fig. 4.13 Scleral-depressed vitreous shaving

Vitreous base vitrectomy is then performed (Fig. 4.13). The chandelier light allows the surgeon to carry out this maneuver without assistance. Scleral-depressed vitrectomy allows peripheral vitreous shaving, which results in a more complete vitrectomy. It is important to accurately remove peripheral vitreous as much as possible, especially in the supero-temporal quadrant from where, in a second step, we will enter with the electrode array into the vitreous cavity through the sclerotomy cut. The presence of residual adhesion of cortical vitreous in this region could induce a stretching of the ciliary bodies during the insertion of the chip into the vitreous cavity with all the unpleasant consequences that might arise (such as marked hypotonia in the postoperative period and subsequent development of choroidal detachment).

If macular epiretinal membrane is present in the region where the array will be located, it is peeled away, and if the patient is aphakic, we will remove any posterior capsule that remains.

In the supero-temporal quadrant, a 5.2 mm straight sclerotomy, with a distance from the limbus calculated according to the axial length-related tables mentioned above, is now performed. To create the sclerotomy, we use first a 15° single edge knife perpendicularly angled to the sclera, being careful not to cut the ciliary body. The use of a narrow and sharp knife is suitable to ensure a full-thickness and full-width incision of the soft and elastic choroid coat. Slightly decreasing intraocular pressure may reduce the resistance felt during choroid cut and make it easier to perform. Then we use a 5.2 mm premeasured angled bevel up to widen the wound and to reduce resistance during insertion of the array (Fig. 4.14).

At this point we can introduce the array into the eye (Fig. 4.15).

The array is grasped on a special "handle" located on the distal end of the array with 20-gauge end-gripping forceps and is inserted into the mid-vitreous cavity with an angle of insertion perpendicular to the sclera. The array is released in the

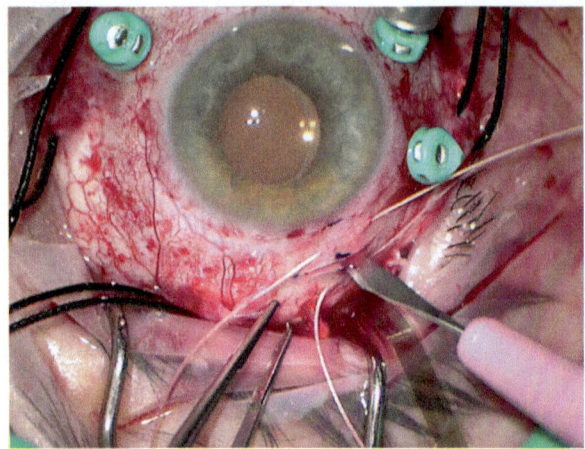

Fig. 4.14 5.2 sclerotomy cut with a 15° single edge knife

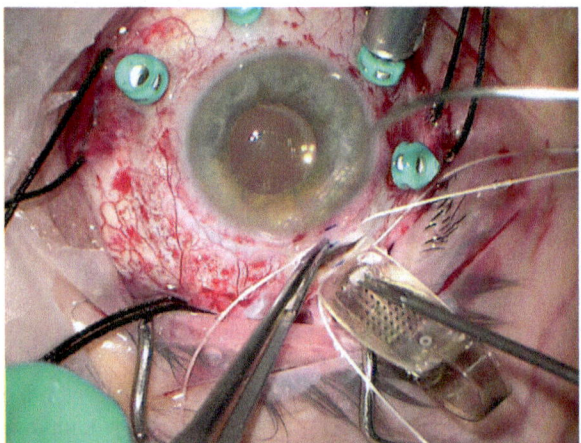

Fig. 4.15 Array insertion through sclerotomy grabbing the array with 20-gauge Eckardt end gripping

mid-vitreous cavity, and the remaining extraocular part of the cable is pushed inside with silicone forceps. Before definitively fixing the array onto the retina, the scleral wound is closed with multiple interrupted 6-0 or 7-0 Vicryl sutures. The stitches on the 5.2 sclerotomy must be given as close as possible to each other, being careful not to damage the cable. This is to avoid future leakage, always keeping in mind that, even with very close stitches, an opening between the inside and outside of the eye will always remain due to the cable passing through the sclera.

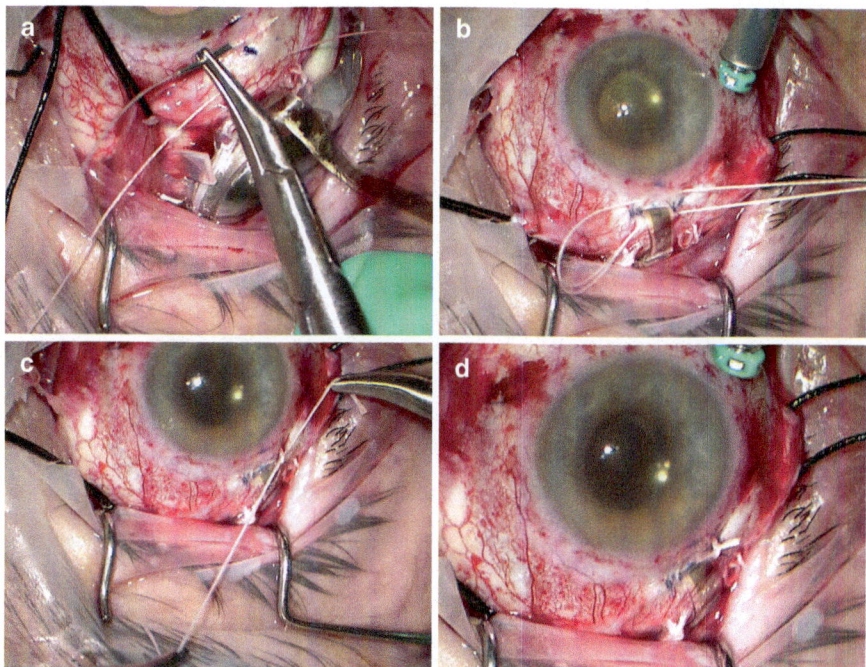

Fig. 4.16 (**a**) Purse-string suture. (**b**) Purse-string suture. (**c**) Purse-string suture. (**d**) Purse-string suture

Sometimes, if leakage persists, a 5-0 Mersilene purse-string suture is placed around the sclerotomy to allow hermetic closure at the electrode cable site and to reduce risk of postoperative hypotony and long-term complications (Fig. 4.16a–d).

If all the previous steps have been performed correctly, the array should fall on the macular region (the initial location of the array is generally nasal of the macula). Next, the surgeon, using intraocular end-gripping forceps, tries to position the array in the ideal location. This should result in the electrode rows being approximately diagonal at 45° to the horizontal meridian and the center of the electrode grid coinciding with the fovea, leaving a small non-electrode portion of the array just touching the optic disc (Fig. 4.17).

If the array appears tilted when placed on the fovea or there is substantial twist in the cable, the surgeon should relocate the extraocular portion of the device to correct the cable angle entering the sclerotomy. When the surgeon is ready to proceed with tacking, he creates another 20-gauge sclerotomy port in the inferonasal quadrant to introduce the tack tool, then he loads the tack into the tack insertion tool (making sure that the tack is in line with the tool shaft), and finally he fixes the array to the retina with a bimanual technique: with one hand (through end-gripping forceps) the surgeon grips the little handle on the array and places it in the ideal

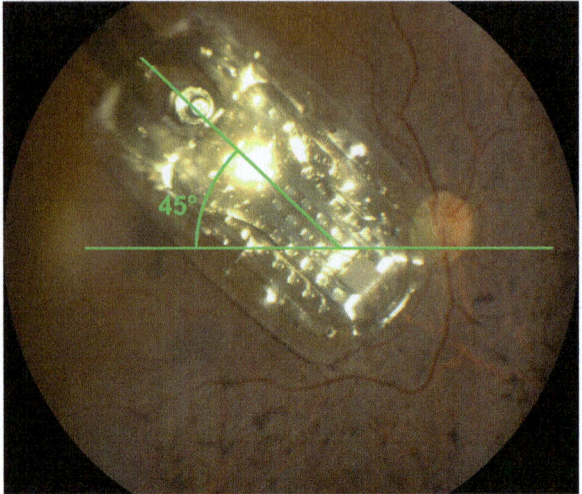

Fig. 4.17 Array ideal position: electrode rows positioned at 45° to the horizontal meridian with the array center coinciding with the fovea

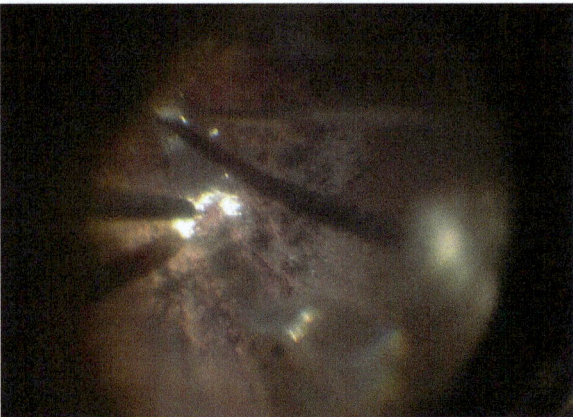

Fig. 4.18 Bimanual array tacking onto the retina

position, while with the other hand (using a special tack insertion tool via the 20-gauge sclerotomy), he proceeds to insert the tack in the dedicated hole located at the root of the array and fixes it into the retina (Fig. 4.18).

During this maneuver, the intraocular pressure must be set at 60 mmHg, and the tack insertion tool must be placed as perpendicular to the retinal surface as possible before inserting the tack into the retina.

Use of chandelier lighting system helps to illuminate the retina and frees the surgeon's second hand, allowing him to perform a bimanual technique.

Phase 4: Closure

If the implant placement is correct, and there are no complications, we proceed to suture the 25- and 20-gauge sclerotomies with 7-0 or 8-0 Vicryl (during the closure phase, infusion line is left in place).

Moreover, to avoid movement and extrusion of the cable, a mattress suture is passed above the cable.

To prevent conjunctival erosion, a piece (approximately 9 mm × 7 mm) of cadaveric human pericardium or equivalent allograft (SJM Pericardial Patch with Encap TM Technology or Biologics Tutopatch by Tutogen Medical GmbH) is fixed above the array cable and the electronic case suture tabs using 7-0 Vicryl absorbable sutures (Fig. 4.19). The 25-gauge infusion trocar is then removed, and the sclerotomy is sutured. Tenon's and conjunctiva are sutured with 8-0 Vicryl (Fig. 4.20), and a subconjunctival injection of 1 cc cefazolin (100 mg) and 1 cc dexamethasone (2 mg) salt solution is given far away from the implant. Finally, an intravitreal injection of 0.1 cc vancomycin (1 mg/0.1 cc) and 0.1 cc ceftazidime (2.25 mg/0.1 cc) is performed (Table 4.1 intraoperative medication).

Phase 5: Intraoperative Implant Testing Procedure

This procedure is not performed as a step in its own right but in conjunction with the four surgical steps. During the implantation procedure, it is important to perform the impedance measurement of the 60 platinum electrodes of the array to verify that no

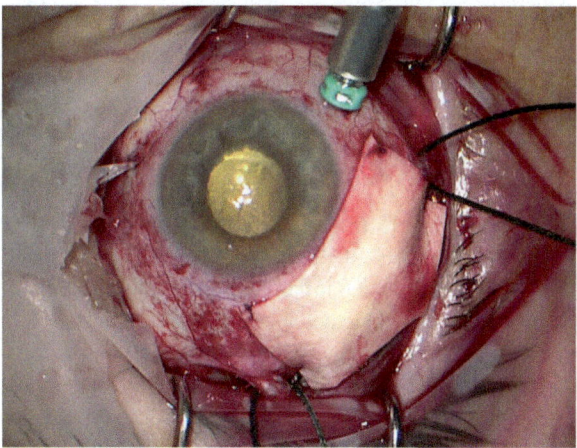

Fig. 4.19 9 × 7 pericardial patch is fixed above the array cable and the electronic case suture tabs using 7-0 Vicryl

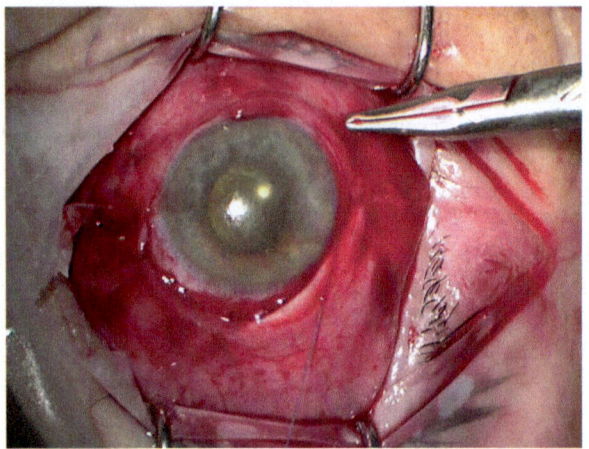

Fig. 4.20 Conjunctiva closure with 8-0 Vicryl

changes or damage of the matrix elements or of the electrical polymer cable have occurred during surgical maneuvers.

There are five intraoperative times when it is recommended to test the system:

1. Impedance measurement in solution
2. Impedance measurement after the extraocular placement (optional)
3. Impedance measurement before intraocular array tacking (optional)
4. Impedance measurement after intraocular array tacking
5. Impedance measurement after the final closure (optional)

In order to perform the intraoperative implant test, we need supplementary equipment provided by Second Sight Medical Products (Fig. 4.21):

1. Argus® II operating room (OR) coil: a radio-frequency (RF) coil that will allow the clinician to monitor the implant safety
2. Argus® II clinician fitting system (CFS): laptop computer that is configured with a dedicated, PC-based software that enables tailoring of the electrical stimulation parameters for the patient, as well as monitoring and troubleshooting of the system

In the operating room, the electrode impedance measurements are performed on demand. To test the functionality of the implant, the external OR coil is placed in close proximity to the implant. Once it has established a good link with the internal coil, the external OR coil communicates the status of the implant to the laptop. The impedance measurement takes less than 30 s. The software will display a color-coded map of impedance values: the lower value, the better the condition of the electrode. In the same condition, for example, if the electrode array is not sufficiently wet with salt solution or if there has been damage to the implant during its manipulation, the impedance measurement could indicate electrodes with high impedance values. In this case, we have to repeat the measurement by ensuring that the chip is well immersed in the salt solution in order to exclude damage to the system.

CFS Laptop

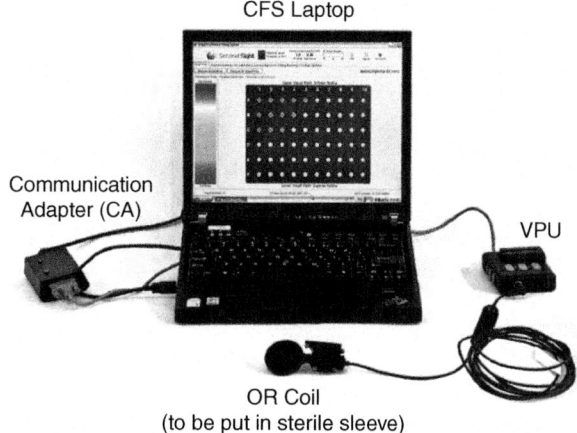

Communication
Adapter (CA)

VPU

OR Coil
(to be put in sterile sleeve)

Fig. 4.21 External equipment composed of CFS laptop, video-processing unit (VPU), OR coil, and communication adapter (CA) (image courtesy of Second Sight Medical Products)

Table 4.2 Pre- and postoperative medication

Preoperative medication	48 h of 500 mg oral antibiotics fluoroquinolone (or equivalent) two times/day
Postoperative medication	14 days of 500 mg oral antibiotics fluoroquinolone (or equivalent) two times/day
	14 days oral steroid prednisolone (or equivalent) 60 mg daily followed by a period of tapering dose
	14 days of topical antibiotic fluoroquinolone (or equivalent) eye drops, one drop four times per day
	14 days topical steroid prednisolone drops 1% (or equivalent), one drop four times daily (continue beyond 2 weeks as needed)
	14 days topical drops atropine 1% (or equivalent), one drop every day

Recommended Pre- and Postoperative Medication Regimen

The patient who receives an Argus® II epiretinal prosthesis is subjected to a regimen consisting of antibiotic and cortisone systemically as well as topically.

For 48 h before surgery, patients are treated with 500 mg of systemic oral antibiotics fluoroquinolone (or equivalent) for two times/day and topical antibiotic fluoroquinolone eye drops (one drop four times/day).

In the postoperative phase, the patient will be administered 14 days of topical antibiotic fluoroquinolone eye drops (one drop four times/day); topical steroid prednisolone eye drops (one drop four times/day), to be continued for a further 2 weeks as needed; and atropine 1% eye drops (one drop daily). Postoperative systemic therapy consists in 14 days of full-dose (1000 mg/day) oral antibiotics fluoroquinolone and 14 days of oral steroid prednisolone (60 mg daily for 2 weeks followed by 8 mg methylprednisolone taper pack, until the pack is finished) (Table 4.2).

Postoperative Management

Postoperative management follows the patient in three distinct and equally important aspects:

1. To calibrate the microchip stimulation parameters customizing them to each patient's need
2. To allow the best integration of the device in the patient's everyday life thanks to specifically designed visual rehabilitation
3. To regularly perform medical examinations of the implanted eye and check the patient's general health

Calibration Phase

Calibration phase refers to the procedure for customizing the video-processing unit (VPU) for use by the subject. Calibration phase takes place over several sessions following implantation of the Argus® implant, and it takes place in the clinic. During the calibration phase, first (array scanning) all 60 electrodes of the microchip are stimulated one by one in order to induce single spots of light and verify which electrodes cause perception and which do not. Each active electrode is stimulated three times and at three different electric strengths increasing each time (at 234 μA, at 452 μA, and at 677 μA). If the patient does not have any perception of light in at least two of the three stimulations at the lowest level, the electrode should be stimulated at the next level. At this point, for each electrode of the microchip, the minimum quantity of electricity necessary to induce a perception of light on the part of the patient (hybrid threshold measurement) is measured. Once the basic electric stimulations have been ascertained, they will be used to produce a video configuration file (VCF) specific to each patient (generate VCF tool) which will be loaded onto the video-processing unit (VPU). The video-processing unit (which serves to transform the video image on the camera into electric stimulations of the retina in real time) will generate the correct and diverse electric stimulations for each patient on the basis of the calibration carried out previously.

Rehabilitation Phase

Once the VPU has been calibrated, the actual rehabilitation begins. In the weeks and months following implantation, subjects will receive training on how to use the Argus® system. The image which patients receive with the Argus® II system is different from the normal image they were used to seeing before their loss of sight. Therefore, there are certain basic concepts and visual abilities which patients will need to acquire in order to use the system efficiently and to integrate these "new" images into daily life.

During the rehabilitation phase, patients will need to learn how to regulate the functions present on the VPU, such as the inversion of the background (black images on a white background or white images on a black background: this should be inverted according to the luminosity of the surrounding environment), the regulation of contrast (vision in black and white or in a range of grays), and the definition of the outlines (patients will be able to choose whether to see only the outline of the object/person visualized).

They will need to learn to identify the spatial position of the phosphenes created by the Argus® II system and to differentiate them from the common phosphenes typical of their retinopathy; they should learn to keep their eyes looking straight ahead in respect to their head; on an axis with the external antenna located on their glasses (in order not to lose the electrical connection between the external system and the internal system), they should learn to move their head and eyes at the same time (patients, once implanted, need to get used to scanning their surroundings using movements of their head and no longer their eyes); and they need to practice recognizing the difference in the signal between black and white objects, recognizing white figures on black backgrounds and vice versa, localizing objects on a table, and localizing points of light which come from windows or doors, to the point when they manage to interpret forms, letters, and numbers.

This process must be supported by a qualified visual rehabilitation specialist who has been specifically trained to conduct the reeducation both in internal and external surroundings as well as using visual function tests which are developed and supplied by the Second Sight Company. These tests include the square localization (to determine the ability of the patient to localize luminous squares on a black background), the direction of motion (to determine the ability of the patient to distinguish the movements of luminous bars on a black background), and the grating visual acuity (to measure the patient's visual acuity in a range between 1.6 and 2.9 logMAR).

This rehabilitation should be carried out both in hospital and at home, and it may last from a few months to 1 year, based on the patient's perseverance and ability.

Eye Checkup Phase

The eye checkup examinations should be carried out regularly, above all immediately after surgery in order to avoid medical complications. The checkups evaluate both the general health of the patient and the condition of the eye. They take into consideration both eyes and include not only a complete examination of the eye but also a series of in-depth instrument checkups. For these we advise:

1. Fundus photo (to evaluate the ideal position of the matrix and its possible rotations or movements) (Fig. 4.22)
2. Optical coherence tomography (OCT) (to evaluate distance between array and retina, a possible morphological modifications of the retinal layers, a possible onset of fibrosis around the tack (de Juan et al. 2013) or of fibrotic adhesions between the chip and the internal surface of the retina, a possible onset of retinal schisis or choroidal folds) (Fig. 4.23)

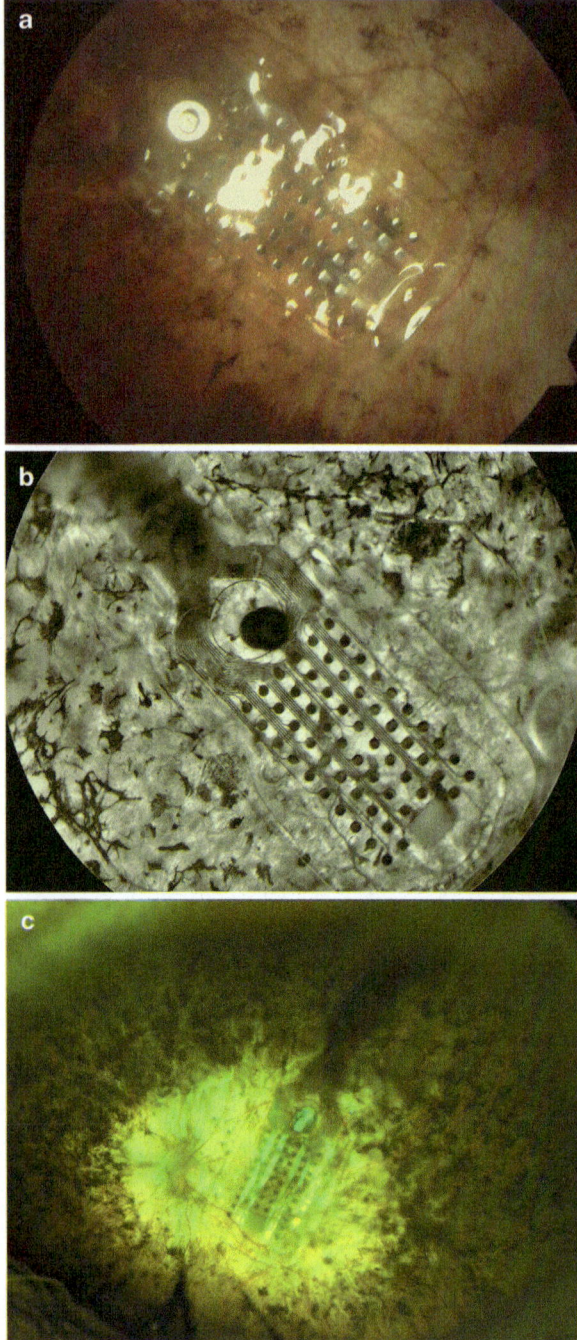

Fig. 4.22 (**a**) Fundus image taken with Topcon DRI OCT Triton, (**b**) autofluorescence imaging taken with the spectral domain Heidelberg Spectralis HRA+OCT, (**c**) A 200° fundus image in a "green separation mode" taken with Optos Daytona

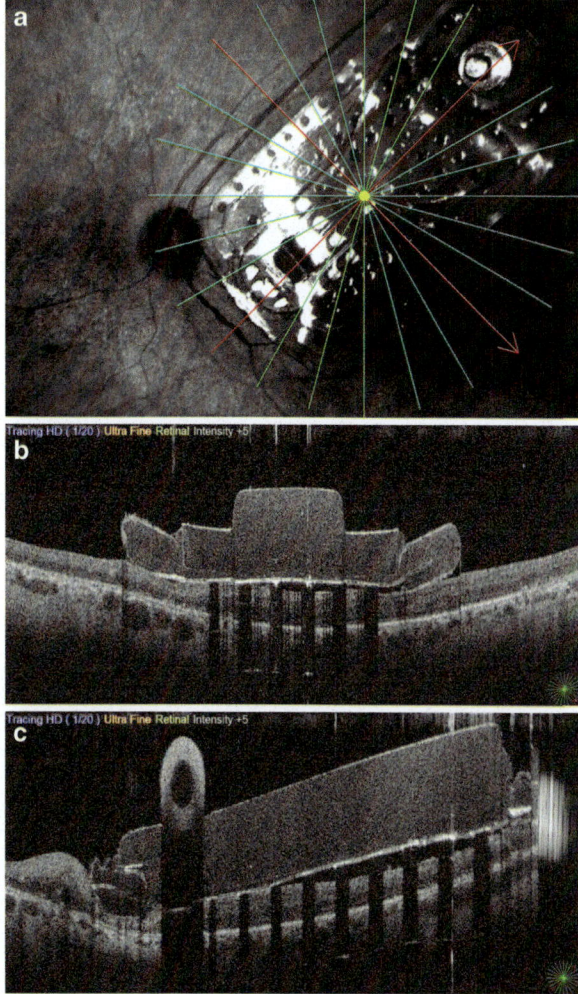

Fig. 4.23 Fundus surface image and cross-sectional images of the retina captured using the NIDEK Optical Coherence Tomography RS-3000 Advance. (**a**) Fundus surface image. The longest electrode row of the array is precisely positioned at 45° to the horizontal meridian with a small non-electrode portion of the array just touching the optic disc. (**b**) Cross-sectional image of the retina-array complex passing through the shorter row of electrodes (composed by six electrodes). The metal electrodes block light from the scanning infrared light source, casting six shadows on the retinal image. (**c**) Cross-sectional image of the retina-array complex passing through the longest row of electrodes (composed of ten electrodes)

3. Goldmann visual field (to evaluate possible changes or improvements of the visual field)
4. B-scan echography (to monitor the course of possible complications such as a choroidal detachment, a retinal detachment, or retinal schisis)

All the data regarding the adverse events were collected. Adverse events were classified as "serious" (if they caused permanent damage or required surgical intervention or hospitalization to prevent permanent impairment) and "nonserious" (if they required noninvasive treatment or resolved spontaneously without any treatment).

Compliance with Ethical Requirements

Stanislao Rizzo and Laura Cinelli declare that they have no conflict of interest. No human or animal studies were performed by the authors for this chapter.

References

de Juan E Jr, Spencer R, Barale PO, da Cruz L, Neysmith J. Extraction of retinal tacks from subjects implanted with an epiretinal visual prosthesis. Graefes Arch Clin Exp Ophthalmol. 2013;251(10):2471–6. https://doi.org/10.1007/s00417-013-2452-y.
Mura M, Bamonte G. Surgical pearls for implantation of the Argus II Retinal Prosthesis 32–34. RETINA Today January/February, 2014.
Second Sight Medical Products, Inc. Argus® II retinal prosthesis system surgeon manual. Sylmar, CA: Second Sight Medical Products, Inc.; 2013. Available at: https://www.accessdata.fda.gov/cdrh_docs/pdf11/H110002C.pdf

Chapter 5
Retinal Prostheses: Clinical Outcomes and Potential Complications

Devon H. Ghodasra, Allen C. Ho, K. Thiran Jayasundera, and David N. Zacks

Introduction

The feasibility of surgical implantation of retinal prostheses for the treatment of retinal degenerations was first demonstrated in animal studies. Early biocompatibility studies showed no serious adverse events, and novel surgical techniques were developed to implant various types of retinal prostheses on or below the retinal surface. While a variety of devices have shown promising outcomes in animal studies, those being implanted in humans are most notable for making technical headway toward clinical application. The recent publication of human clinical trials with long-term outcome and safety data has confirmed the exciting progress in visual prosthesis research.

Clinical Outcomes

Early experiences with retinal prostheses have shown promising results in restoring sight to the blind, but as with any investigational device, patient safety and device reliability are of paramount concern. The first retinal prosthesis to obtain regulatory approval, the Argus II Retinal Prosthesis System (Second Sight Medical Products,

D.H. Ghodasra, M.D. • K. Thiran Jayasundera, M.D. • D.N. Zacks, M.D., Ph.D. (✉)
Ophthalmology and Visual Sciences, University of Michigan, Kellogg Eye Center,
1000 Wall Street, Ann Arbor, MI 48105, USA
e-mail: devonghodasra@gmail.com; thiran@med.umich.edu; davzacks@med.umich.edu

A.C. Ho, M.D.
Clinical Retina Research Unit, Wills Eye Hospital, Retina Service,
840 Walnut Street, Suite 1020, Philadelphia, PA 19107, USA
e-mail: acho@midatlanticretina.com

© Springer International Publishing AG 2018
M.S. Humayun, L.C. Olmos de Koo (eds.), *Retinal Prosthesis*, Essentials in
Ophthalmology, https://doi.org/10.1007/978-3-319-67260-1_5

Inc., Sylmar, CA, USA), has shown an acceptable long-term safety profile as compared to glaucoma drainage devices and retinal tacks (Gedde et al. 2009; Lankaranian et al. 2008; Ang et al. 2010; Abrams et al. 1986). One study of the 12-month outcomes of six patients from a single center showed no complications that required additional surgery (Rizzo et al. 2014). The 3-year results of the Argus II clinical trial showed an acceptable rate of serious adverse events (SAEs) and nonserious adverse events (non-SAEs) (Ho et al. 2015). SAEs are defined as complications that require medical or surgical intervention to prevent permanent injury. Non-SAEs are those that may be observed or for which treatment is noninvasive. Thirty subjects were implanted with the Argus II between June 2007 and August 2009 at ten centers in the United States and Europe (Ho et al. 2015). Implant safety was examined at years 1 and 3. The majority of patients, 66.7% at year 1 and 63.3% at year 3, had no device- or surgery-related SAEs. The most common SAEs were conjunctival erosion or dehiscence, hypotony, presumed endophthalmitis, retinal tack dislocation requiring re-tacking, and retinal tear or detachment. Other SAEs include corneal opacity, infective keratitis, and corneal melt. Nonserious adverse events include epiretinal membrane, conjunctival congestion, ocular pain, hypotony, suture irritation, choroidal detachment, uveitis, retinal thickening, and vitreous hemorrhage, among others.

Patients are at greatest risk for both serious and nonserious adverse events during the early postoperative period. At year 3, 61% Argus II SAEs and 53% of non-SAEs had occurred within the first 6 months after implantation. Vigilant monitoring during follow-up appointments is critical during this period.

Certain implanted patients may be at increased risk for multiple or recurrent complications. The Argus trial showed that events were clustered within patients as 55% of all SAEs at 3 years occurred in only three subjects (10%). Furthermore, the few delayed complications observed after 6 months were usually a part of cascades or recurrences of events. Complications associated with retinal prosthesis are frequently related. The development of one such complication may increase the risk of future complications. For example, the presence of hypotony or conjunctival erosion may allow the ingress of microorganisms into the vitreous cavity from the ocular surface and may increase the risk of endophthalmitis. Further study is needed to identify those patients that are most at risk for recurrent complications.

As clinical experience with retinal implants grows, devices have shown good long-term reliability. The Argus II System has been shown to be very reliable and stable. Twenty-nine out of 30 implanted subjects still had functioning devices after 3 years. A single patient was explanted due to complication management rather than device failure. Seven patients had elective surgical repositioning of the array to improve function, but no devices have been explanted due to nonfunctioning.

Postoperative care and the management of complications in patients undergoing retinal prosthesis are critical in achieving successful outcomes. In addition to the typical risks associated with standard intraocular surgery, retinal prosthesis surgery raises new challenges from the unique aspects of the implantation procedure. Preoperative planning and modified surgical techniques may help reduce the risks of certain complications. Patients require close follow-up and vigilant monitoring of any symptoms that may alert of an impending complication. Early detection aids in early rehabilitation, which can minimize long-term sequelae.

Complications and Management Strategies

Conjunctival Erosion

Conjunctival erosion or dehiscence is the most common complication arising with retinal prosthesis implantation (Ho et al. 2015; Humayun et al. 2012). In the Argus II clinical trial, 13.3% of subjects had conjunctival erosion, and 10.0% had conjunctival dehiscence defined as a serious adverse event. Three patients (10%) had conjunctival erosion or dehiscence defined as a nonserious adverse event. Conjunctival disruption typically occurs over the raised profile of suture tabs of the extraocular component of the device. Conjunctival erosion and dehiscence are often heralded by ocular irritation or pain, conjunctival injection, tenderness to palpation, or mucoid discharge (Fig. 5.1). Examination of the suspected area of erosion may reveal overlying conjunctival hyperemia, visible sclera, or exposed suture/prosthesis (Fig. 5.2).

While early identification is most critical, several pre- and intraoperative strategies may reduce the likelihood of conjunctival problems. A preoperative risk assessment should note previous ocular surgery which can cause conjunctival scarring and identify thin or poorly mobile conjunctiva on preoperative examination. Any history

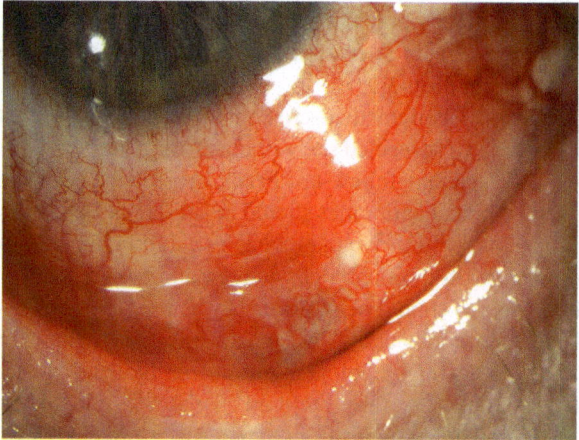

Fig. 5.1 Early conjunctival erosion over the device suture Table 3 months after implantation treated with removal of eroding Mersilene suture, placement of pericardial graft, and conjunctival closure

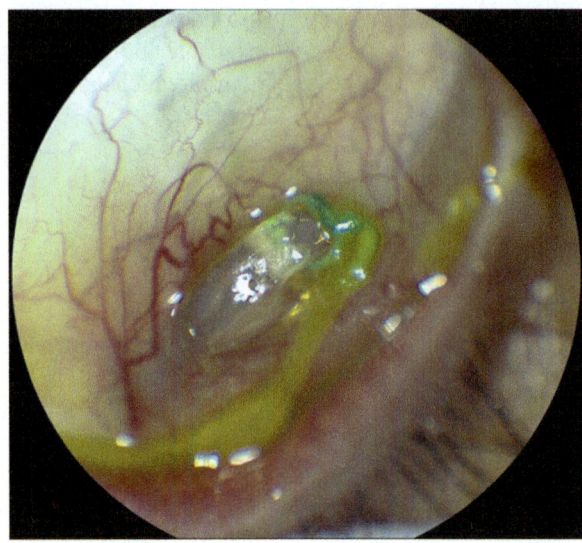

Fig. 5.2 Late conjunctival erosion and exposed device suture tab leading to eventual device explantation

of strabismus or extraocular muscle surgery should be identified. One Argus II patient with a history of large muscle recession had conjunctival erosion because the device coil could not be placed under the lateral rectus. Intraoperatively, the electronics case, array cable, and suture tabs should be adequately covered with an allograft such as processed pericardium. The Tenon's membrane should be closed with absorbable suture prior to meticulous conjunctival closure. For suturing the scleral buckle, nylon suture may be preferred over braided Mersilene polyester sutures, which may contribute to erosion. All permanent sutures should be rotated posteriorly to lower knot profiles.

Ideal management of conjunctival erosion involves early identification. Mild injection and irritation at a suspected site without erosion can be treated with aggressive lubrication and frequent follow-up. Frank erosion or dehiscence should be managed surgically. Topical antibiotics should be used until the patient can return to the operating room for closure. Wound revision should include adequate exposure of the offending area with thorough debridement and release of any areas of traction. All irritating sutures should be removed. If the buckle and coil are secure and well encapsulated, suture tabs can be removed if necessary. Exposed areas should be recovered with sufficient homologous scleral or pericardial patch graft, over which conjunctiva is then carefully reclosed. If there is not sufficient remaining conjunctiva for closure, an autograft from the fellow eye may be used.

Conjunctival erosion is a significant risk for the lifetime of a retinal prosthetic device. Implanted patients should be vigilant in promptly reporting any new symptoms of foreign body sensation, pain, tearing, or discharge to their surgeon.

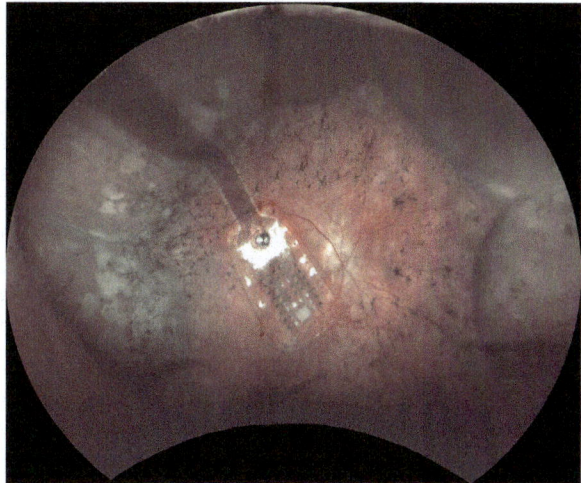

Fig. 5.3 Choroidal detachment secondary to hypotony presenting on postoperative day 3

Hypotony

Postoperative hypotony is one of the more common complications of retinal pros-thesis surgery. Conservative management may be appropriate in some cases, but surgical invention with wound revision is the definitive treatment. In the Argus II clinical trial, hypotony was defined at intraocular pressure less (IOP) than 5 mmHg (Humayun et al. 2012). Four patients (13.3%) had hypotony defined as a serious adverse event requiring treatment to prevent injury, and seven patients (23.3%) had hypotony defined as nonserious that was managed with observation or noninvasive methods. Postoperative hypotony typically occurs within 6 months of implantation, but cases have been reported after 12 months (Ho et al. 2015). Acute postoperative hypotony is typically due to inadequate closure of sclerotomies but less commonly may be due to damage to the ciliary body. The case of late postoperative hypotony in the clinical trial was attributed to migration of the device after broken sutures. Nevertheless, there may be a lifetime risk of hypotony due to the presence of the open channel of the array cable (Humayun et al. 2012). Hypotony may be asymp-tomatic or can cause eye pain and discomfort. Ophthalmic examination may reveal corneal decompensation, shallowing of the anterior chamber, anterior chamber cell and flare, or ciliochoroidal detachment, either serous or hemorrhagic (Fig. 5.3). Seidel testing with fluorescein should be performed for all patients with hypotony or suspected leaks.

Prevention of postoperative hypotony is best achieved by meticulous sclerotomy closure, especially the superotemporal sclerotomy around the array cable. Adequate closure of sclerotomies at the end of the case is facilitated by proper initial wound construction. The sclerotomy for the array cable should be straight as opposed to a chevron shaped or curved, which may cause cable and wound puckering. When closing, mattress sutures with long scleral passes increase vector forces in re-apposing wound edges. Each sclerotomy should be dried and carefully checked for leakage. Any small amount of oozing from the wound should be addressed, as spontaneous resolution should not be assumed. Some surgeons advocate fluid-air exchange, suggesting that the surface tension effect of an air bubble can help reduce wound leaks. Partial thickness scleral flaps analogous to trabeculectomy surgery and sealants such as fibrin glue have been used but are not standard practice.

Management of postoperative hypotony depends on duration of hypotony and any associated signs. If no other serious adverse events are present, observation for up to 2 weeks with pressure patching and close follow-up can be adequate. Persistent hypotony or unimproved anterior chamber flattening should prompt return to the operating room for further inspection and re-suturing of sclerotomies. Small or stable choroidal effusions may also be observed, but quickly enlarging or appositional choroidal effusions warrant immediate reoperation. In the interim results from the Argus II clinical trial, two of three patients with hypotony had stabilization of IOP with intraocular silicone oil tamponade (Humayun et al. 2012).

Endophthalmitis

Infectious endophthalmitis is a rare occurrence in typical vitrectomy surgery, occurring in approximately 1 in 3000 cases (Hu et al. 2009; Shimada et al. 2008; Scott et al. 2008). There are several aspects unique to retinal prosthesis implantation, however, that may increase the risk of endophthalmitis. The higher risk of conjunctival erosion and the persistent channel of the array cable both open the barrier between the intraocular cavity and external environment. The prolonged time of surgery of retinal implantation as compared to standard vitreoretinal procedures may also contribute to increased risk. In the long-term results from the Argus II clinical trial, 3 out of 30 implanted patients (10%) had culture-negative endophthalmitis (Ho et al. 2015). In the single-study center of six patients, there were no cases of endophthalmitis (Rizzo et al. 2014). Endophthalmitis is typically associated with increasing eye pain and photophobia. Examination may reveal conjunctival injection, severe anterior chamber reaction with hypopyon or fibrin, and vitreous cell and haze (Figs. 5.4 and 5.5).

The most important step to reducing the risk of postoperative endophthalmitis is preoperative povidone iodine prep and sterile technique. The retinal implant and device cable should also be rinsed prior to implantation, and all efforts should be made to avoid contact with exposed lashes. Topical and subconjunctival antibiotics should be used postoperatively to cover Gram-positive and Gram-negative bacteria. Oral antibiotics are used per device protocol for 1–2 weeks. After the protocol in the Argus II clinical trial was changed to include prophylactic intravitreal antibiotics at the end of the case, no additional cases of endophthalmitis were reported (Ho et al. 2015). Contributory risks such as hypotony and conjunctival erosion should be

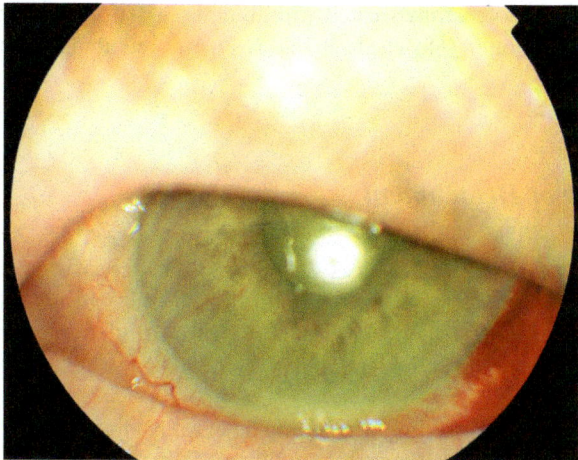

Fig. 5.4 Endophthalmitis presenting with pain, conjunctival injection, subconjunctival hemorrhage, engorged iris vessels, and hypopyon 5 weeks after implantation

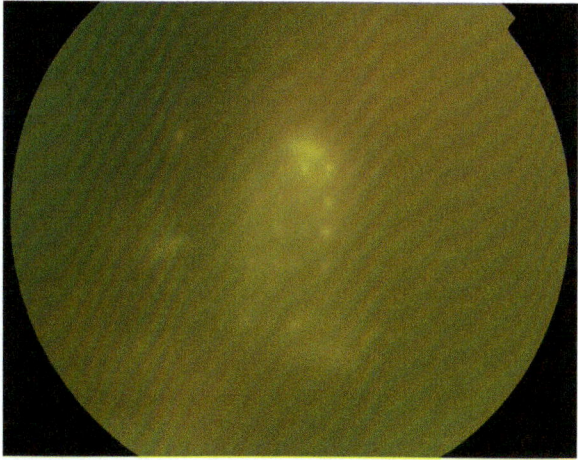

Fig. 5.5 Vitritis and hazy view of the fundus in the preceding patient with endophthalmitis

identified early and corrected. The early identification of presumed endophthalmitis is also critical to preserving successful outcomes. Warning signs and symptoms of endophthalmitis should be reviewed at each follow-up examination, and patients should be instructed to call immediately with concerns.

As in all intraocular surgery, suspected endophthalmitis should be considered an ophthalmic emergency. Vitreous aspiration and culture should be performed. Intravitreal antibiotics typically given are vancomycin 1 mg/0.1 mL and ceftazidime 2.25 mg/0.1 mL. Due to its effective vitreous penetration, an oral fluoroquinolone should be considered for 7–14 days. All cases of endophthalmitis in the Argus II clinical trial were successfully treated with intravitreal, subconjunctival or topical, and systemic antibiotics (Ho et al. 2015). No cases required explantation of the device.

Retinal Tear or Detachment

Retinal tear and detachment are less common serious adverse events noted after retinal prosthesis implantation. In 30 Argus clinical trial patients, one had retinal tear, and two had retinal detachments (Ho et al. 2015). Both cases of retinal detachment occurred 5–6 months after surgery and were treated with surgical intervention (Fig. 5.6).

Several intraoperative techniques should be employed to reduce the risk of this complication. First, some surgeons recommend that triamcinolone acetonide be used to highlight the vitreous and allow for more accurate and safer shaving of the vitreous base in both the superotemporal and inferotemporal quadrants where the array and the tack, respectively, will be inserted. Second, excessive traction on the retina should be avoided. Since the vitreous cortex is very adherent in some patients with RP, the hyaloid frequently cannot be detached anterior to the mid-periphery. Third, macular epiretinal membranes may be peeled to improve contact between the array and the retina, but internal limiting membrane peeling should not be performed to avoid the risk of macular hole. Fourth, prophylactic 360° endolaser retinopexy is not recommended as this may cause necrosis of the retina, which is

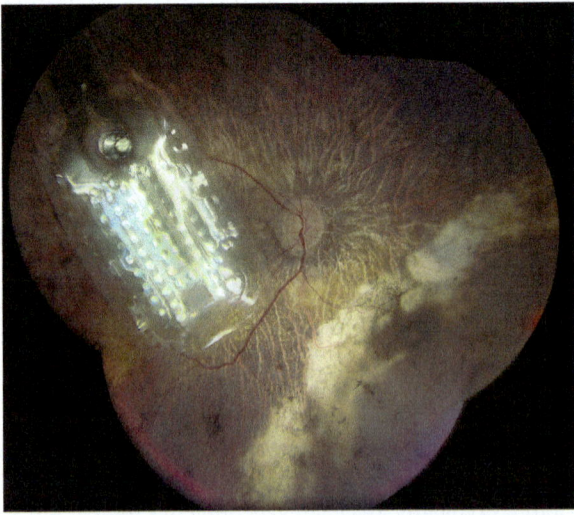

Fig. 5.6 Laser demarcation of suspected rhegmatogenous retinal detachment in the inferonasal quadrant noted on routine follow-up 2 weeks after device implantation

already thin and atrophic. Lastly, careful examination of the periphery with scleral depression at the end of the case allows immediate detection and treatment of intra-operative retinal breaks.

Retinal tears and detachments may be treated with standard surgical techniques. All vitreous adhesions and tractional membranes should be fully released. Any reti-nal breaks should be well treated with confluent retinopexy. Laser retinopexy may be safely used without altering electrode functioning, but care should be taken to ensure laser is applied away from the intraocular portions of the device. Both intra-ocular gas (SF6 and C3F8) and silicone oil may be used for tamponade without affecting the retinal prosthesis. As with other complications, the symptoms of reti-nal tear and detachment should be discussed with each patient during follow-up to assure prompt diagnosis.

Nonserious Adverse Events

Like most serious adverse events, nonserious adverse events or minor complications typically arise within the first 6 months after implantation. These device- and procedure-related complications may include ptosis, macular edema, epiretinal membrane, uveitis, and elevated intraocular pressure.

Macular Complications

Retinal thickening and cystoid macular edema are commonly seen after intraocular surgery, including vitrectomy. Retinal prosthesis implantation may have increased risk of macular edema because of increased postoperative inflammation compared to standard vitreoretinal surgery and unique tractional aspects arising from prosthe-sis contact with the retinal surface. In the Argus II clinical trial, 16.7% of patients had retinal thickening with cystoid macular edema, and 13.3% had retinal thicken-ing without cystic changes (Ho et al. 2015). Cystoid macular edema is characterized by breakdown of the blood-retinal barrier with accumulation of fluid in the inner nuclear and outer plexiform layers, producing a petaloid pattern. Oral and topical steroids are used as part of the typical regimen to reduce postoperative inflamma-tion. The Argus II clinical trial protocol used topical prednisolone and oral pred-nisolone for 2 weeks followed by methylprednisolone (Medrol) taper pack. For recurrent or residual macular edema, topical nonsteroidals (ketorolac) and/or dor-zolamide may be used as needed. If not improving, a 1-month course of oral pred-nisone (0.5 mg/kg to start, then tapered weekly) can be considered. While it should generally be treated, the effect of prolonged or persistent edema on electrode func-tioning is unknown. Cases have even been reported in which array-retina apposition improved after incidence of macular edema, resulting in improved electrode functioning.

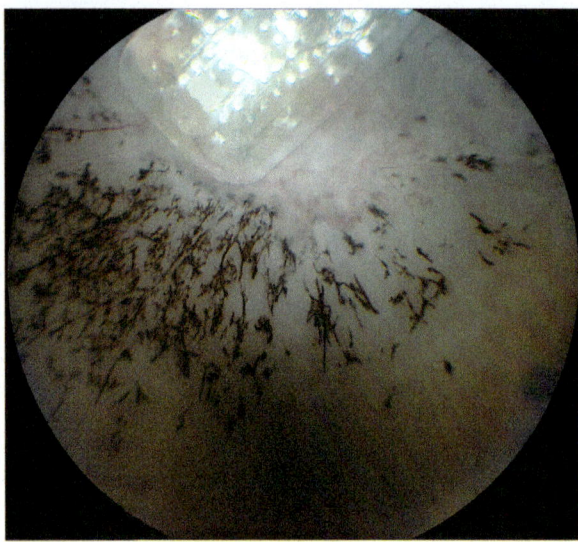

Fig. 5.7 Dense epiretinal membrane near the device array causing tractional retinal detachment 6 weeks after implantation

Epiretinal membranes typically form from residual vitreous cortex left during vitrectomy or in response to postoperative inflammation. More specifically in retinal prosthesis implantation, array contact with the retinal surface may also contribute (Fig. 5.7). Of the 30 Argus II clinical trial patients, 11 (36.7%) developed a postoperative epiretinal membrane. Both epiretinal membrane and macular edema can be followed with optical coherence tomography. Postoperative epiretinal membrane formation is typically observed without treatment, but its effect on long-term retinal prosthesis functioning needs further study.

Elevated Intraocular Pressure

While hypotony is the more common pressure issue, patients undergoing retinal prosthesis surgery have several risk factors for developing postoperative elevated intraocular pressure. Increased intraocular pressure is observed in approximately one-third of patients following standard vitreous surgery (Han et al. 1989; Gedde 2002; Costarides et al. 2004; Desai et al. 1997). The majority of pressure elevation after standard vitrectomy is due to secondary open-angle glaucoma and includes causes such as inflammation or corticosteroid response. Retinal prosthesis patients may have increased intraocular inflammation compared to patients undergoing standard vitreoretinal procedures that are shorter and require less manipulation. Argus II patients also receive higher and prolonged doses of topical and oral steroids, which may place them at risk for steroid response glaucoma. Increased intraocular pressure typically occurs 2–6 weeks after initiation of steroid treatment. The risk of postoperative intraocular pressure elevation may also be higher in retinal prosthesis patients due to elements of the scleral buckle. For standard vitreoretinal procedures such as retinal detachment repair, combined procedures involving vitrectomy and scleral buckle have been shown to increase the risk of developing postoperative elevated pressure (Han et al. 1989). The placement of an encircling scleral buckle is known to temporarily reduce the outflow facility of the eye. In the Argus clinical trial, 2 out of 30 patients (6.7%) developed postoperative elevated intraocular pressure.

All patients should be instructed about the warning signs of elevated intraocular pressure during standard postoperative counseling. At each follow-up examination, intraocular pressure should be assessed, ideally with the Goldmann applanation tonometry. Accurate pressure monitoring may sometimes be difficult in the early postoperative period due to corneal epithelial defects or edema. Upon identification of elevated pressure, any secondary factors such as increased inflammation should be appropriately managed. Intraocular pressure may be controlled with topical medications, including beta-blockers (e.g., timolol), alpha agonists (e.g., brimonidine), and carbonic anhydrase inhibitors (e.g., dorzolamide) as needed and as tolerated. Pilocarpine should be avoided if possible. Systemic oral carbonic anhydrase inhibitors (e.g., acetazolamide) may also be used as needed. Patients with known glaucoma or angle abnormalities should be vigilantly monitored and treated early for pressure fluctuations.

Attentive monitoring of intraocular pressure is necessary in all patients undergoing retinal prosthesis surgery.

Uveitis

Surgical manipulation may result in alterations of the blood-aqueous and blood-retinal barriers, leading to vulnerability to inflammation in the early postoperative period. Protein leakage and cellular reaction in the aqueous and vitreous humor are manifested as cell and flare or vitreous haze. Some degree of inflammation is to be expected after any complex surgical procedure such as retinal prosthesis implantation, but early identification of an excessive inflammatory response is needed to ensure absence of infection and to help promote normal wound healing. The most important initial step in addressing atypical postoperative inflammation is identifying noninfectious uveitis from infectious endophthalmitis. While differentiating the two may sometimes be challenging, features suggesting an infectious etiology include significant pain, intense conjunctival injection, fibrin or hypopyon, and timing 3–10 days after surgery. Any suspicion of inflammation from an infectious etiology should be treated as endophthalmitis and managed as previously discussed. Delayed onset endophthalmitis from fungal or atypical bacteria such as *P. acnes* is especially challenging in differentiating from noninfectious chronic postoperative uveitis. Five patients (16.7%) with noninfectious uveitis were identified in the 3-year results of the Argus clinical trial (Ho et al. 2015).

After microbial infection has been ruled out, noninfectious postoperative uveitis can be addressed. Typical signs of uveitis include ciliary flush, anterior chamber cell or flare, keratic precipitates, and vitreous haze or cell. Intraocular pressure should be measure and is typically low or normal but may become elevated from uveitic glaucoma. Mild anterior chamber reaction can be treated with topical prednisolone acetate 1% (Pred Forte). Once inflammation is improving, the steroid can be tapered by one drop per day every week and then discontinued once all cells have disappeared from the anterior chamber. Intermediate and posterior uveitis is treated with oral steroids or sub-Tenon's steroid injection. Patients are typically started on oral prednisone 40–60 mg per day. With improvement, prednisone is tapered by 5–10 mg weekly depending on response. Sub-Tenon's injection of triamcinolone 40 mg/mL may also be considered in patients with cystoid macular edema and intermediate or posterior uveitis but is contraindicated in patients with steroid-responsive intraocular pressure. Cycloplegic agents such as cyclopentolate 1% or atropine 1% should be given to prevent synechiae and reduce photophobia.

The risk of postoperative uveitis is typically reduced with an appropriate postoperative steroid regimen. Topical and oral steroids should be used as recommended by the retinal prosthesis protocol and tapered as inflammation permits. Any patient with history of uveitis should be identified preoperatively as intraocular surgery may cause prolonged and severe postoperative inflammation. Implantation should be delayed in any patient with active uveitis. These patients should be treated appropriately and remain quiet without any evidence of active inflammation, or rebound for at least 3 months before implantation should be considered. Any patient with a history of uveitis may warrant preoperative pulse dose oral steroids immediately prior to implantation.

Postoperative uveitis is expected after retinal prosthesis surgery, but excessive inflammation may lead to additional complications such as macular edema, elevated intraocular pressure, or tractional retinal membranes. Appropriate management of disproportionate or rebound uveitis can preserve good outcomes in patients undergoing retinal prosthesis implantation.

Conclusion

Retinal degenerations such as retinitis pigmentosa were previously one of the major causes of untreatable blindness. New treatment paradigms such as gene therapy and retinal prostheses have the potential to revolutionize the management of these patients. Clinical trials of various retinal prostheses are well underway, and the most examined implant, the Argus II Retinal Prosthesis System, has already shown favorable long-term safety data. The risk of serious and nonserious adverse events for retinal prosthesis implantation is comparable to other intraocular procedures. Long-term reliability and device failure rate are excellent. Despite promising overall results, early experiences have also identified certain challenges and complications associated with novel parts of the surgical procedure. In addition to standard risks associated with vitreoretinal surgery, the implantation procedure has increased risks of complications such as conjunctival erosion, hypotony, endophthalmitis, and retinal tear or detachment. In some instances, the risk of complications may be reduced with modified techniques to implantation protocol. More importantly, vigilant monitoring for early potential complications is critical to successful postoperative management. Data have shown that long-term sequelae can be minimized with appropriate medical and surgical management.

Acknowledgments The authors would like to thank Dr. Janet L. Davis and Dr. Ninel Z. Gregori for providing the fundus photographs of their patients with retinal detachment (Fig. 5.6) and epiretinal membrane (Fig. 5.7) at the Bascom Palmer Eye Institute, Miami, FL. The authors would also like to thank Dr. Lyndon daCruz for providing anterior segment and fundus photographs of his patient with endophthalmitis (Figs. 5.4 and 5.5) at the Moorfields Eye Hospital, London, UK.

Compliance with Ethical Requirements Devon H. Ghodasra, David N. Zacks, and K. Thiran Jayasundera declare that they have no conflict of interest. Allen C. Ho is a past consultant for Second Sight Medical Products, Inc. No human or animal studies were carried out by the authors for this chapter.

References

Abrams GW, Williams GA, Neuwirth J, McDonald HR. Clinical results of titanium retinal tacks with pneumatic insertion. Am J Ophthalmol. 1986;102(1):13–9.

Ang GS, Varga Z, Shaarawy T. Postoperative infection in penetrating versus non-penetrating glaucoma surgery. Br J Ophthalmol. 2010;94(12):1571–6. https://doi.org/10.1136/bjo.2009.163923.

Costarides AP, Alabata P, Bergstrom C. Elevated intraocular pressure following vitreoretinal surgery. Ophthalmol Clin N Am. 2004;17(4):507–12. https://doi.org/10.1016/j.ohc.2004.06.007.

Desai UR, Alhalel AA, Schiffman RM, Campen TJ, Sundar G, Muhich A. Intraocular pressure elevation after simple pars plana vitrectomy. Ophthalmology. 1997;104(5):781–6.

Gedde SJ. Management of glaucoma after retinal detachment surgery. Curr Opin Ophthalmol. 2002;13(Table 1):103–9. https://doi.org/10.1097/00055735-200204000-00009.

Gedde SJ, Schiffman JC, Feuer WJ, Herndon LW, Brandt JD, Budenz DL. Three-year follow-up of the tube versus trabeculectomy study. Am J Ophthalmol. 2009;148(5):670–84.

Han DP, Lewis H, Lambrou FH Jr, Mieler WF, Hartz A. Mechanisms of intraocular pressure elevation after pars plana vitrectomy. Ophthalmology. 1989;96(9):1357–62.

Ho AC, Humayun MS, Dorn JD, et al. Long-term results from an epiretinal prosthesis to restore sight to the blind. Ophthalmology. 2015;122(8):1547–54. https://doi.org/10.1016/j.ophtha.2015.04.032.

Hu AYH, Bourges JL, Shah SP, et al. Endophthalmitis after pars plana vitrectomy. A 20- and 25-gauge comparison. Ophthalmology. 2009;116(7):1360–5. https://doi.org/10.1016/j.ophtha.2009.01.045.

Humayun MS, Dorn JD, Da Cruz L, et al. Interim results from the international trial of second sight's visual prosthesis. Ophthalmology. 2012;119(4):779–88.

Lankaranian D, Reis R, Henderer JD, Choe S, Moster MR. Comparison of single thickness and double thickness processed pericardium patch graft in glaucoma drainage device surgery: a single surgeon comparison of outcome. J Glaucoma. 2008;17(1):48–51. https://doi.org/10.1097/IJG.0b013e318133fc49.

Rizzo S, Belting C, Cinelli L, et al. The Argus II retinal prosthesis: 12-month outcomes from a single-study center. Am J Ophthalmol. 2014;157(6):1282–90.

Scott IU, Flynn HW, Dev S, et al. Endophthalmitis after 25-gauge and 20-gauge pars plana vitrectomy: incidence and outcomes. Retina. 2008;28(1):138–42. https://doi.org/10.1097/IAE.0b013e31815e9313.

Shimada H, Nakashizuka H, Hattori T, Mori R, Mizutani Y, Yuzawa M. Incidence of endophthalmitis after 20- and 25-gauge vitrectomy. Causes and prevention. Ophthalmology. 2008;115(12):2215–20.

Chapter 6
Retinal Prostheses: Functional Outcomes and Visual Rehabilitation

Gislin Dagnelie

Introduction

The quality of prosthetic vision is extremely poor. Most of us are surrounded by screens with millions of pixels in rich color and can hardly imagine a visual world presented in low contrast and without meaningful color. The resolution of a retinal prosthesis may be specified as 6 × 10 (Argus II) to 38 × 40 (Alpha IMS), but in reality there are no discernible pixels at all, and the implants provide at best blurry shape and movement information. And yet some recipients of these implants demonstrate surprising ability to interact with the visual world around them in ways that seem inconceivable when we look at realistic simulations of what they are seeing. This simple reflection teaches us two important facts:

1. Even minimal visual information can be helpful to a person who has been functionally blind for years.
2. The human visual cortex is remarkably good at learning how to interpret this very limited information.

In this chapter, we will consider how this is possible and how we can assess and improve prosthetic visual performance.

The question how many dots are needed to convey an image goes back at least to the dawn of television transmission, but for visual prostheses this question was first seriously examined in the Normann lab at the University of Utah in the 1980s, in the context of design proposals for a cortical visual prosthesis. Cha and colleagues studied the minimum number and density of dots required for reading (Cha et al. 1992c), visual acuity sufficient for standard print (Cha et al. 1992a), and wayfinding in an

G. Dagnelie, Ph.D.
Department of Ophthalmology, Johns Hopkins University School of Medicine, Johns
Hopkins Hospital, Wilmer Woods 358, 1800 Orleans Street, Baltimore, MD 21287, USA
e-mail: gdagnelie@jhmi.edu

© Springer International Publishing AG 2018
M.S. Humayun, L.C. Olmos de Koo (eds.), *Retinal Prosthesis*, Essentials in
Ophthalmology, https://doi.org/10.1007/978-3-319-67260-1_6

indoor maze (Cha et al. 1992b). For all three tasks, a grid of 25 × 25 dots with 4 arc-min spacing presented foveally was found to yield good results, albeit that a mini-fied image was required for optimal mobility, projecting a 30° visual field onto the 1.7° grid. All these simulations were carried out in normally sighted individuals, with the assumption that future prosthesis recipients would all be previously sighted and thus have a fully developed central visual system.

As several teams began to design retinal prostheses, it became clear that implants with 625 electrodes would not be feasible in the near future, and additional simula-tions were carried out to determine what tasks could be accomplished with feasible electrode numbers. The Johns Hopkins group compared simulations with 4 × 4, 6 × 10, and 16 × 16 dots for a variety of clinical and daily tasks (Hayes et al. 2003)—tumbling E, Lea symbols, MNRead (Legge et al. 1989), recognizing household objects, pouring, and cutting with scissors—and for both real and virtual wayfind-ing tasks (Dagnelie et al. 2007). An important finding of these studies was that a few of the simplest tasks could be carried out with just 4 × 4 dots, and all could be learned with 6 × 10. These findings informed the choices by Second Sight for its first (Argus 16, 4 × 4 electrodes) and second (Argus II, 6 × 10 electrodes) implant designs and several other groups based their designs on similar considerations. Subsequent simulations of face recognition (Thompson et al. 2003) and continuous text reading (Dagnelie et al. 2006a) indicated that 16 × 16 dot resolution could be adequate for more complex visual tasks.

Figure 6.1 shows several of the "pixelized" patterns presented to sighted subjects using a video headset. When viewing these stationary patterns, it is important to bear in mind that these subjects derived additional information from the temporal changes in the patterns as the camera was scanned across the scene and that in most cases performance could be improved with practice.

In retrospect, these early simulations, and dozens of similar studies performed by groups around the world to project how well future implant recipients might be able to accomplish visual tasks, suffered from a major flaw: They all assumed that the images perceived by implant wearers would consist of a grid of regularly spaced dots, similar to the output of a dot matrix printer. While that assumption was in part supported by reports of small round phosphenes, obtained during intraoperative tests in blind volunteers, some acute tests indicated that phosphenes could be irregu-larly shaped (Rizzo et al. 2003). Acute tests with a row of electrodes also indicated that elongated compound shapes were seen, rather than a row of individual dots. This lack of resolution down to individual dots, even for electrodes separated by 2° (~550 μm), has been confirmed in all chronic retinal implants to date: Images are described as blurred shadows, as though each dot is "smeared out" by the simultane-ous activation of neighboring electrodes; this effect may be attributed to mutual interference of cellular activation patterns in the inner retina caused by extensive reorganization of neuronal connectivity in the later stages of retinal degeneration (Jones and Marc 2005).

Figure 6.2 shows pairs of images for two hand-eye coordination tests carried out in our lab, originally by normally sighted and low-vision observers and more recently by Argus II implant users. The first test, the so-called checkerboard task,

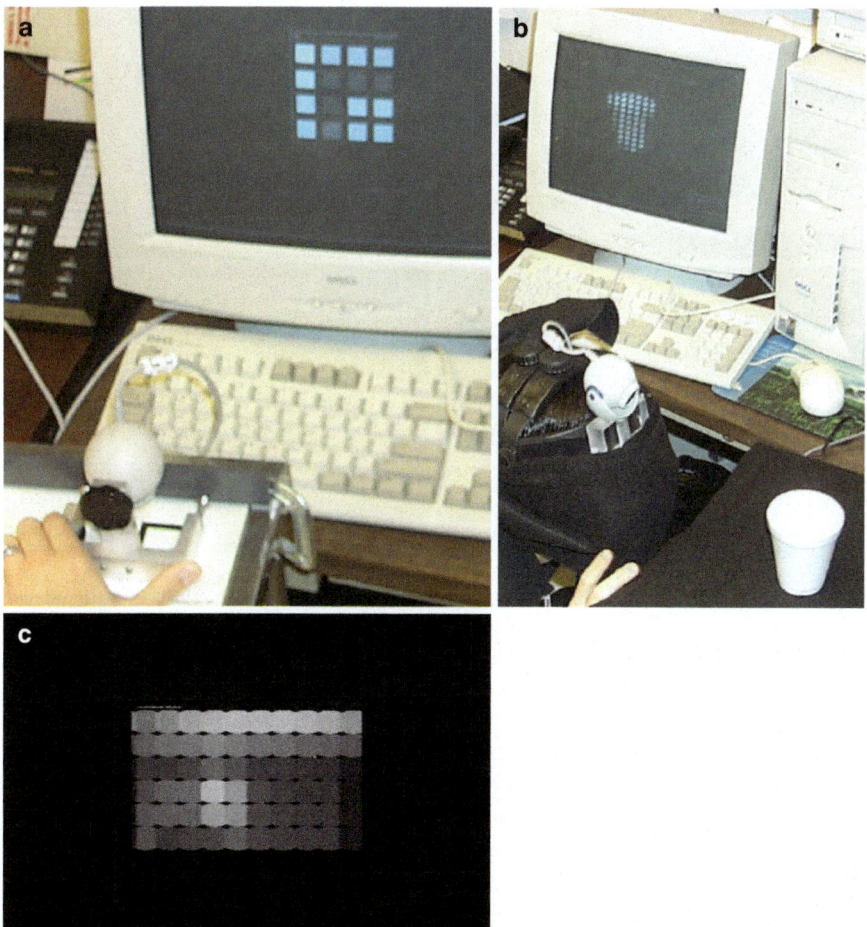

Fig. 6.1 Three simulations developed in the author's laboratory: (**a**) Percept of a partial Lea symbol using a 4×4 electrode retinal prosthesis. (**b**) Percept of a white Styrofoam cup within the field of view of a 16×16 electrode retinal prosthesis. (**c**) Percept of the view into a room, with a ceiling light and a window, as seen with a 6×10 retinal prosthesis

required the subject to locate a small number of white squares within a white frame and then cover these squares with black checkers (Dagnelie et al. 2006b); the images in Fig. 6.2a/b show the video capture by the subject's head-worn camera and the image presented in the head-worn goggles, respectively. In the second test, the "maze-tracing" task, subjects placed a stylus on a black dot inside a white circle on a touchscreen and then had to trace a white line with one of more angles to reach a solid circle marking the end of the maze (Mueller et al. 2007); the images in Fig. 6.2c/d show the starting circles and stylus captured by the subject's camera and the image presented to the subject—notice that the position of the stylus can still be inferred from the interruption in the white ring.

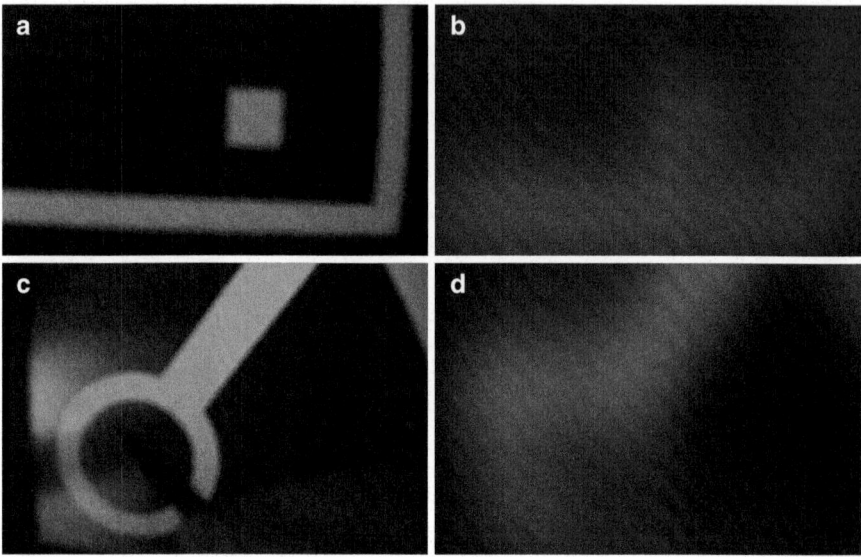

Fig. 6.2 Views of detail of the board during the "playing checkers" activity (**a/b**) and of the screen during a "maze-tracing" task (**c/d**). (**a**) and (**c**) show raw images as captured by the subject's head-worn video camera; (**b**) and (**d**) show the images as they are thought to appear to the retinal implant wearer

Early simulations did not do justice to another crucial aspect of prosthetic vision with an external camera, i.e., the role of head vs. eye movements in scanning the scene: In normal vision, and in a retinal prosthesis with intraocular image capture, the image projected onto the retina, and thus the information sent to the central visual system, will shift in response to an eye movement, but the oculomotor system sends a corollary discharge of the eye movement command to the central visual system (Duhamel et al. 1992), so the image shift is anticipated and perceived as a stationary scene. With a head-mounted camera, on the other hand, this closed-loop system is interrupted: The electrodes stimulating the retina move with the eye, and the compensatory signal to the central visual system causes the eye movement to be perceived as a shift. This requires the prosthesis wearer to learn to keep the eyes steady and perform camera scanning movements with the head. While the still images in Fig. 6.2 cannot show this, an eye tracker inside the video headset worn by our sighted subjects was used to shift the image in register with eye movements, allowing us to verify whether they could learn to keep the eyes still. We found that they indeed learned to do so (Wang et al. 2008) and eventually perform at levels close to free-viewing conditions (Kelley et al. 2004), thus providing confidence that retinal implant wearers would learn to do so as well.

Based on the most realistic simulations and despite severe limitations of today's prosthesis systems, it appears, therefore, that retinal implant wearers should be able to accomplish simple visual tasks. There are several additional factors, however, that could further restrict patient performance: the distance from the implanted electrodes to the target cells, the condition of the inner retina, the quality of the electrical signal transduction from the implant to the retina, unintended activation of retinal ganglion cell axons in the retinal nerve fiber layer, and gradual deterioration of the implant or the retina, whether related to long-term stimulation or merely to aging. On the other hand, it is important to remember that the human central visual system is capable of extremely sophisticated pattern detection and recognition, especially with well-targeted rehabilitation and practice. Without the ingenuity of the visual cortex, the perseverance of the implant users, and the support of dedicated rehab specialists, many of the results reported below would not be possible.

Functional Outcomes

Patients receiving retinal implants will generally be those with end-stage inherited retinal degenerations. This implies that they have had good, or at least useful, vision in youth, and sometimes for decades, but they all have gone through a period where they were functionally blind, with at best some light perception or projection. A retinal implant restores some functionality, and the best way to assess this is to follow the crude hierarchy:

- Light perception (telling daylight from night or room lights on from off)
- Light projection (where the light is coming from)
- Light movement (direction in two dimensions)
- Detecting contrast (borders, outlines)
- Spatial resolution (two dots/bars)
- Crude hand-eye coordination
- Shape discrimination
- Monocular depth cues (size, parallax)
- Functions requiring detail vision, such as reading, face recognition, fine motor tasks, etc.—well beyond the capabilities of current retinal implants

Reading the reports on clinical trials with various retinal implants, one finds this same progression of visual tasks and functional assessments (Mahadevappa et al. 2005; Benav et al. 2010; Ayton et al. 2014; Fujikado et al. 2011; Roessler et al. 2009), and one can think of this hierarchy as framework for a prosthetic vision curriculum; in fact, all groups working with implant recipients use a similar framework. Some projects, notably the German Epiret 3 project and the suprachoroidal implant programs in Japan and Australia, have had fewer implanted patients and shorter time periods and have therefore not tested all aspects listed above. For this reason, and because we are most familiar with the Argus II studies, this overview will limit itself primarily to results published for the Argus II. Another reason to look at only one system in depth is that there appears to be a general consensus that the two best-documented implant systems, the Alpha IMS and the Argus II, yield very similar functional performance (Stronks and Dagnelie 2014; Zrenner 2013; Ho et al. 2015).

Light perception is not assessed as a separate test but rather verified as part of the initial system "fitting," i.e., determining the minimum electrical charge at which phosphenes can be elicited, either at a single electrode or through a combination of multiple adjacent electrodes. During a similar procedure, the dynamic range of the implant is determined by scoring perceived brightness as a function of electrical charge, limited either by the patient's comfort level or by the charge limits set by the electrode materials or implant electronics. Once a brightness vs. charge characteristic has been obtained for all functional electrodes, the electronics of the prosthesis system are set to allow a direct conversion from external illumination to perceived brightness; note that either the camera system or the internal electronics must perform the automatic gain adjustment required for operation of the system at widely varying absolute illumination levels. Only after the system electronics have been properly tuned can the hard work of "prosthetic seeing," i.e., interpreting phosphene stimulation patterns, begin. Most patients will initially describe their prosthetic vision as "seeing flashes," and only gradually will these flashes become organized into movement and patterns, as the visual system works to detect their meaning.

Once the implant wearer has learned to reliably detect the presence of light, the next step is to detect where the light is coming from. In the Argus II training sequence, this is done through an exercise called square localization (Ahuja et al. 2011): A white square subtending ~5° is presented in a random location on a touchscreen in front of the subject, at a distance of ~40 cm, and the subject's task is to touch the perceived location of the square on the screen; automatic verbal feedback regarding the closeness and correct direction is provided by the software—e.g., "close; it was higher and right"—after each trial, and a distribution of relative touch deviations is saved at the end of each run of 40 trials. Published results from the Argus II feasibility study show that, at 1 and 3 years after implantation, 90% of subjects were significantly more accurate in their localization (Ho et al. 2015) and that the variability for most of them was at most one-third, with the system on compared to system off (Ahuja et al. 2011); the only exceptions were three subjects whose remaining vision allowed them limited localization.

The localization of a light source requires the prosthesis wearer to scan the camera across the light and determine where the source is in reference to the head. Pointing to the light source requires translation from a head-centered to a body-centered frame of reference. An additional complicating factor is eye position: Similar to the effect of gaze shifts mentioned above, the location of a stimulus perceived by the wearer of an implant with an external camera depends on the direction of gaze (Sabbah et al. 2014), but this location may shift over time depending on the proprioceptive feedback received. This was demonstrated by Barry and Dagnelie (2016), who intentionally provided a "gaze" offset to several Argus II wearers by shifting the portion of the wide-field camera image that was presented to the implant. The study indeed found an adaptation process, but it was much slower than the adaptation observed in sighted individuals wearing prisms (Held and Hein 1958).

Having a central gaze direction or a body-centered frame of reference is less important in determining the direction of a bar stimulus moving across a touchscreen, the stimulus used in the so-called direction of motion test (Dorn et al. 2013), although the response does require the subject to trace the perceived direction on the screen. But as long as the head is held vertical, the perceived and traced direction should closely match the stimulus direction. During the clinical trial, directions were randomized, and 80 trials were presented in each run, with verbal feedback similar to that in the square localization test following each trial. A distribution of error angles was saved at the end of each run. Even though this task might seem easy, the time during which the stimulus was visible as the bar crossed the field of view of the implant was short, and the accuracy was limited by the resolution of the implant. For this reason, only ~60% of subjects performed significantly better with the system on compared to system off (Ho et al. 2015); in fact, in addition to the same three subjects who could perform the task with the system turned off, ten subjects performed at the chance level with the system turned on (Dorn et al. 2013).

As a simple but demonstrably reliable measure of spatial resolution, the Argus II trial used a grating visual acuity test (Bittner et al. 2005), adapted for use on a monitor screen at 40 cm. Square-wave gratings with 100% contrast, ranging in width from 40 to 800 arcmin (20/800 to 20/16,000 or 1.6 to 2.9 logMAR, in 0.1 logMAR steps), were presented in one of four orientations (horizontal, vertical, diagonal left, or diagonal right) for up to 5 s, and subjects indicated the perceived direction by pressing one of four response buttons. Due to the limited extent and resolution of the implant, this test required rapid scanning in different directions for the Argus II wearers to make a reliable choice, so most implant users were unable to meet the strict statistical criteria for reliable detection at adjacent spatial frequencies: An interim study found that 7 of 28 subjects had repeatable resolution thresholds ranging from 1.8 to 2.9 logMAR, while none had measurable resolution with the system off (Humayun et al. 2012). In the latest study report (Ho et al. 2015), the number of implant users with measurable grating acuity was 14 out of 29 after 1 year and 9 out of 27 after 3 years.

To address the task of shape recognition/discrimination, Argus II clinical trial participants were invited to join a letter identification task. The alphabet was separated into three groups based on shape characteristics: simple (L,T,E,J,F,H,I,U), intermediate (A,Z,Q,V,N,W,O,C,D,M), and complex (K,R,G,X,B,Y,S,P). All characters were presented in white on a black background, with 2.9 logMAR font size. Among 21 participants, correct percentage levels with the system on for the three letter groups were 72 ± 25%, 55 ± 27%, and 52 ± 29%, respectively; performance with the system off was no better than chance (da Cruz et al. 2013). Six subjects continued the test with smaller characters, in 0.1 logMAR steps. Finally, four of these six subjects were challenged to "read" short words, at their preferred font size and with their eyes patched. They were given up to 60 s per character and managed to successfully identify 7–10, 5–9, and 4–9 out of 10 two-, three-, and four-letter words, respectively. Clearly, this is not a practical reading alternative for braille or speech output, but it does confirm that some retinal prosthesis wearers can recognize complex shapes, including short words. A similar report has appeared about at least one recipient of the multi-photodiode array (MPA) subretinal implant (Retina Implant AG, Reutlingen, Germany), the predecessor of the Alpha IMS (Zrenner et al. 2011).

Several tests of visually guided behavior in the laboratory have been reported for Argus II users. Two of these formed part of the clinical trial (Ho et al. 2015): In the "line task," subjects followed a white line on the floor that either ran straight for 18 ft. or made a 90° left or right turn midway; successful completion required the subject to follow the line to the end; six trials were performed, two in each configuration, in pseudorandom order. The success rate was close to $70 \pm 6\%$ across 28 subjects at 1 and 3 years after implantation with the system on and was at chance with the system off. In the "door task," a 2.5 × 6 ft. rectangular felt "door" was suspended against a contrasting wall, in one of two positions; subjects had to locate it from across a 20 ft. room, walk toward it, and touch it. Success rates were lower (~$53 \pm 6\%$ at 1 and 3 years after implantation), mostly because of near misses and because large objects of the same brightness are hard to locate at close range: Subjects tend to use edge information and thus may touch the wall on the wrong side of the edge.

Other visually guided behavior was reported for smaller numbers of Argus II users in the laboratory. Twenty-one subjects performed the maze test mentioned above (Fig. 6.2c/d); feedback tones were provided so the subject could hear when they correctly touched the starting and end points of the maze. Deviation from the maze pattern was significantly less with the system on as compared to off, but time to complete the task was much longer, not surprising since most subjects haphazardly ran their hand across the screen in the system off condition. In a separate study, six Argus II recipients grasped an object placed at random positions on the table in front of them. In this study, in addition system on and off, a condition called "scrambled" was presented, in which the mapping of the electrodes was randomized, greatly hampering precision but still allowing crude localization. Interquartile ranges for success in the on, scrambled, and off conditions were 67–95%, 42–95%, and 0–50%, respectively, confirming that hand-eye coordination is improved by activation and by correct mapping of the implant electrodes.

All activities listed above were carried out in the clinic, under tightly controlled conditions, and thus were not necessarily representative of activities in everyday life. For this reason, the Argus II clinical trial added three activities under real-world conditions that could vary somewhat from center to center: sock sorting, walking direction discrimination, and sidewalk tracking. In the sock sorting task (Fig. 6.3), a pile of 30 socks—ten white, ten gray, ten black—of the same size and material was placed on a table in front of the subject, on either a high, white or black felt, or low, bare table, wood or gray, contrast background. Subjects were asked to sort the socks into three piles of like color and identify each pile when finished. Subjects performed at chance with the system off and significantly above chance ($73 \pm 23\%$) with the system on, especially on the high-contrast background; error rates were highest for the gray socks, with some subjects performing at chance on the bare table. Interestingly, several subjects commented in subsequent visits that they were now sorting laundry at home.

Two additional tasks were also performed significantly better with the system on than the system off. In an outdoor task, 27 subjects had to follow a curved border between a grass and light-colored sidewalk, without stepping onto the grass or

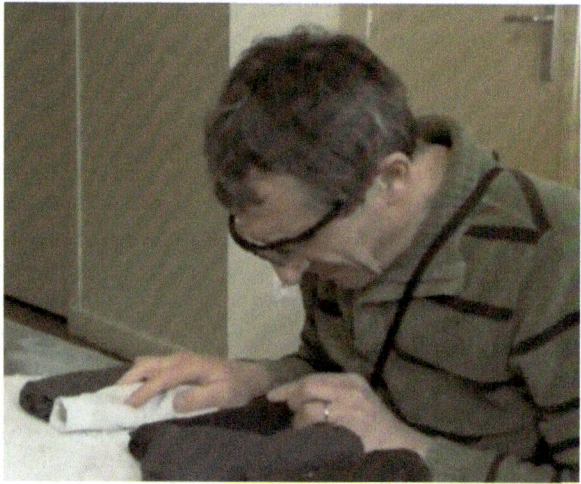

Fig. 6.3 Argus II implant user performing the sock sorting activity

straying more than 3 ft. from the border; errors along a 20 ft. trajectory were counted as the score. In an indoor task, subjects observed two assistants as they took turns passing in front of them at 10 ft. distance and after each of 40 such passages had to indicate whether the person walked left to right or right to left; assistants wore dark tee shirts for contrast against the white backdrop and socks to avoid auditory cues. A few subjects performed above chance with the system off, probably due to remaining auditory information; all performed above chance with the system on.

Patient-Reported Outcomes

As in other areas of clinical research, self-reported outcomes such as visual functioning questionnaires (VFQs) and quality-of-life (QoL) instruments are of great importance when assessing the feasibility or success of retinal implants. After all, even if the objective improvements in function are modest by the standards of normal vision, the differences compared to functional blindness may have a profound impact on the implant wearer. This impact is readily apparent in interviews with Argus II wearers and participants in other retinal prosthesis trials that have been distributed through the media, but an important question is whether the impact can be confirmed using the psychometrically validated self-report instruments (Massof and Rubin 2001) that have increasingly been adopted over the past decade. VFQs in different languages have undergone rigorous calibration using Rasch analysis and are now in use in many clinical trials. Unfortunately, these VFQs are aimed at populations with mild to moderate vision loss and thus do not lend themselves to use in retinal prosthesis wearers—even the simplest activities queried in these instruments would be rated as either "impossible" or "not applicable"; an additional complication is that some activities, like "telling time," may be answered as though they are carried out without using vision and thus be rated much easier than they would be if use of vision were explicitly required.

The Argus II clinical trial used the Massof Activity Inventory (AI) (Massof et al. 2007) and vision-related quality-of-life (VisQoL) (Duncan et al. 2016) instruments to estimate the impact of the implant on participants' vision use and quality of life, respectively. Most of the goals in the AI were rated as not applicable, both at baseline and during follow-up administrations, and many of those that did get scored yielded inconsistent changes; the simplest explanation for this is that this comprehensive categorical list of daily visual activities does not cover retinal implant users' very limited visual ability. Interestingly, three of the six VisQoL subscales—injury, life, and roles—showed a significant response among Argus II implant users who had indicated at baseline that blindness affected their quality of life, with two additional subscales, assistance and activity, showing a positive trend (Duncan et al. 2016). This is understandable, since QoL instruments are not dependent on a particular vision level but rather on the impact of vision change, at any level.

Visual Rehabilitation

Prosthetic vision rehabilitation has many parallels with low-vision rehabilitation in cases of severe visual impairment, but there are two fundamental differences: (1) Prosthetic vision differs in many ways from native vision, as we have seen above; (2) implant users generally are accomplished in blindness skills, and most have received extensive blind rehabilitation. What does remain similar, on the other hand, is the need for concrete rehabilitation goals, allowing the patient and therapist to work on skills development that will make it possible to reach those goals. For these reasons, rehabilitation workers engaging retinal implant recipients need to combine unique skills. They should be experienced in blind rehabilitation, because they have to build on those blindness skills to make the implant an additional tool—it does not replace the blindness skills but augments them. But rehab workers also have to have a thorough understanding of the technology, an attentive ear to what the user is experiencing, and a creative mind to envisage solutions that will make it possible for the user to accomplish valued tasks.

Before and during the rehabilitation process, it is important to observe implant wearers' use of vision, both native and artificial, for any effects of the implant on their daily lives. During the Argus II clinical trial, this need led to the development of the Functional Low-Vision Observer-Rated Assessment (FLORA) (Geruschat et al. 2015, 2016), consisting of three sections: an interview querying the implant wearer for specific changes in activities of daily living (ADL), independence, or social interactions that may be attributed to the implant; an observation of the implant wearer demonstrating specific skills such as indoor orientation in space, perception and direction of light, movement, and objects, object localization and manipulation, and outdoor orientation and wayfinding; and a summary by the rehab specialist conducting the interview and making the observations. Out of 35 activities evaluated in 26 clinical trial participants, 24 were performed significantly better with the system on, as compared to off. The report and recordings submitted by the rehab specialist were reviewed by two outside experts and scored for a net benefit or loss attributable to the device; they concluded that no patients had an overall negative outcome of the implant, and only six had not experienced a benefit.

For the Argus II clinical introduction, SSMP developed a several practical tools such as a magnetic board with black and white sides, and different white and black shapes to be placed on the board, and a kit with three-dimensional objects that can be observed and manipulated to improve image understanding and hand-eye coordination. These instruction tools are used by the rehab specialists during face-to-face training but also are used for practice between training sessions. Home visits and practice in the community are other important aspects of the training program, allowing rehab specialists to observe and advise implant wearers toward more effective use of their restored vision and integration of its use into their blindness skill set.

Toward Improved Functional Outcomes

Over the next few years, improvements in functional outcome can be expected in three important areas:

Image information for prosthesis wearers: At the present time, images presented to retinal implant wearers with external cameras only undergo basic processing, such as adjustment to external luminance and contrast, and video inversion. Laboratory tests have been carried out, either in simulations or with implant wearers, that demonstrate the feasibility of edge enhancement, object localization and recognition, localization of faces, and selection based on distance or temperature using specialized stereo and thermal cameras, respectively. Formal results in implant wearers have not yet appeared in the peer-reviewed literature, but can be expected in the next few years, as can prototype input devices and software performing these functions.

Assessment of visual performance: As indicated above, most visual functioning questionnaires query the respondents about visual activities that cannot be performed with prosthetic vision and therefore are not capable of measuring self-reported visual performance; this is true both at baseline and at follow-up or comparing system on and system off performance. In recent years, a VFQ has been developed that can assess functioning in the ultralow vision range (Dagnelie et al. 2014; Jeter et al. 2016). The use of such a questionnaire for accurate assessment of self-reported visual performance is not limited to retinal implant wearers: Outcomes are reliable in native ULV as well as in prosthesis wearers, and similar benefits can be expected for novel treatment modalities such as gene therapy in patients with rudimentary vision from Leber congenital amaurosis.

Quality of rehabilitation programs: Retinal implants are just starting their development, and the number of rehabilitation specialists who have had the opportunity to work with these patients is small. They have had the opportunity to exchange experiences in online collaborations, conference calls, and a recent conference of Argus II experts (Ghodasra et al. 2016). Further improvements can be expected as a new set of standardized performance assessments for activities of daily living (ADL), developed in parallel with the ULV-VFQ, will become available. Such standardized assessments exist for patients with slightly better visual abilities (Finger et al. 2014), and a similar assessment for individuals with ultralow vision is currently being calibrated (ULV-ADL (Dagnelie et al. 2015)). As the number of wearers of Argus II and other retinal implants grows, so will the number and experience of rehab specialists, as well as the range of rehabilitation programs and tools. This will be important to both patients and clinicians: The success of retinal implants will critically depend on the strength of the rehabilitation program.

Compliance with Ethical Requirements Gislin Dagnelie is a consultant to Second Sight Medical Products and is also named as an inventor on several patents related to the Argus II. No human or animal studies were performed by the author for this chapter.

References

Ahuja AK, Dorn JD, Caspi A, McMahon MJ, Dagnelie G, Dacruz L, Stanga P, Humayun MS, Greenberg RJ. Blind subjects implanted with the Argus II retinal prosthesis are able to improve performance in a spatial-motor task. Br J Ophthalmol. 2011;95(4):539–43.

Ayton LN, Blamey PJ, Guymer RH, Luu CD, Nayagam DA, Sinclair NC, Shivdasani MN, Yeoh J, McCombe MF, Briggs RJ, Opie NL, Villalobos J, Dimitrov PN, Varsamidis M, Petoe MA, McCarthy CD, Walker JG, Barnes N, Burkitt AN, Williams CE, Shepherd RK, Allen PJ, Bionic Vision Australia Research C. First-in-human trial of a novel suprachoroidal retinal prosthesis. PLoS One. 2014;9(12):e115239. https://doi.org/10.1371/journal.pone.0115239.

Barry MP, Dagnelie G. Hand-camera coordination varies over time in users of the Argus((R)) II retinal prosthesis system. Front Syst Neurosci. 2016;10:41. https://doi.org/10.3389/fnsys.2016.00041.

Benav H, Bartz-Schmidt KU, Besch D, Bruckmann A, Gekeler F, Greppmaier U, Harscher A, Kibbel S, Kusnyerik A, Peters T, Sachs H, Stett A, Stingl K, Wilhelm B, Wilke R, Wrobel W, Zrenner E. Restoration of useful vision up to letter recognition capabilities using subretinal microphotodiodes. Conf Proc IEEE Eng Med Biol Soc. 2010;2010:5919–22.

Bittner A, Bowie H, Chow AY, Dagnelie G, Group AS. Repeatability of the grating acuity test in advanced retinitis pigmentosa (RP). Invest Ophthalmol Vis Sci. 2005;46:ARVO E-abstr #517.

Cha K, Horch K, Normann RA. Simulation of a phosphene-based visual field: visual acuity in a pixelized system. Ann Biomed Eng. 1992a;20:439–49.

Cha K, Horch KW, Normann RA. Mobility performance with a pixelized vision system. Vis Res. 1992b;32(7):1367–72.

Cha K, Horch KW, Normann RA, Boman DK. Reading speed with a pixelized vision system. J Opt Soc Am A. 1992c;9(5):673–7.

da Cruz L, Coley BF, Dorn J, Merlini F, Filley E, Christopher P, Chen FK, Wuyyuru V, Sahel J, Stanga P, Humayun M, Greenberg RJ, Dagnelie G. The Argus II epiretinal prosthesis system allows letter and word reading and long-term function in patients with profound vision loss. Br J Ophthalmol. 2013;97(5):632–6. https://doi.org/10.1136/bjophthalmol-2012-301525.

Dagnelie G, Barnett D, Humayun MS, Thompson RW Jr. Paragraph text reading using a pixelized prosthetic vision simulator: parameter dependence and task learning in free-viewing conditions. Invest Ophthalmol Vis Sci. 2006a;47(3):1241–50.

Dagnelie G, Walter M, Yang L. Playing checkers: detection and eye-hand coordination in simulated prosthetic vision. J Mod Opt. 2006b;53:1325–42.

Dagnelie G, Keane P, Narla V, Yang L, Weiland J, Humayun M. Real and virtual mobility performance in simulated prosthetic vision. J Neural Eng. 2007;4(1):S92–101.

Dagnelie G, Jeter PE, Adeyemo K, Rozanski C, Nkodo AF, Massof RW. Psychometric properties of the PLoVR ultra-low vision (ULV) questionnaire. Invest Ophthalmol Vis Sci. 2014;55(ARVO E-abstr):2150.

Dagnelie G, Geruschat D, Massof RW, Jeter PE, Adeyemo O. Developing a calibrated ultra-low vision (ULV) assessment toolkit. Optom Vis Sci. 2015;92(AAO E-abstr):E-abstr #155252.

Dorn JD, Ahuja AK, Caspi A, da Cruz L, Dagnelie G, Sahel JA, Greenberg RJ, McMahon MJ. The detection of motion by blind subjects with the epiretinal 60-electrode (Argus II) retinal prosthesis. JAMA Ophthalmol. 2013;131(2):183–9. https://doi.org/10.1001/2013.jamaophthalmol.221.

Duhamel JR, Colby CL, Goldberg ME. The updating of the representation of visual space in parietal cortex by intended eye movements. Science. 1992;255(5040):90–2.

Duncan JL, Richards TP, Arditi A, da Cruz L, Dagnelie G, Ho AC, Olmos de Koo LC, Sahel J-A, Stanga PE, Thumann G, Wang Y, Dorn JD, Greenberg RJ, AIS G. Improvements in vision-related quality of life in blind patients implanted with the Argus II epiretinal prosthesis. Clin Exp Optom. 2016;100(2):144–50.

Finger RP, McSweeney SC, Deverell L, O'Hare F, Bentley SA, Luu CD, Guymer RH, Ayton LN. Developing an instrumental activities of daily living tool as part of the low vision assessment of daily activities protocol. Invest Ophthalmol Vis Sci. 2014;55(12):8458–66. https://doi.org/10.1167/iovs.14-14732.

Fujikado T, Kamei M, Sakaguchi H, Kanda H, Morimoto T, Ikuno Y, Nishida K, Kishima H, Maruo T, Konoma K, Ozawa M. Testing of semichronically implanted retinal prosthesis by suprachoroidal-transretinal stimulation in patients with retinitis pigmentosa. Invest Ophthalmol Vis Sci. 2011;52(7):4726–33.

Geruschat DR, Flax M, Tanna N, Bianchi M, Fisher A, Goldschmidt M, Fisher L, Dagnelie G, Deremeik J, Smith A, Anaflous F, Dorn J. FLORA: phase I development of a functional vision assessment for prosthetic vision users. Clin Exp Optom. 2015;98(4):342–7. https://doi.org/10.1111/cxo.12242.

Geruschat DR, Richards TP, Arditi A, da Cruz L, Dagnelie G, Dorn JD, Duncan JL, Ho AC, Olmos de Koo LC, Sahel JA, Stanga PE, Thumann G, Wang V, Greenberg RJ. An analysis of observer-rated functional vision in patients implanted with the Argus II Retinal Prosthesis System at three years. Clin Exp Optom. 2016;99(3):227–32. https://doi.org/10.1111/cxo.12359.

Ghodasra DH, Chen A, Arevalo JF, Birch DG, Branham K, Coley B, Dagnelie G, de Juan E, Devenyi RG, Dorn JD, Fisher A, Geruschat DR, Gregori NZ, Greenberg RJ, Hahn P, Ho AC, Howson A, Huang SS, Iezzi R, Khan N, Lam BL, Lim JI, Locke KG, Markowitz M, Ripley AM, Rankin M, Schimitzek H, Tripp F, Weiland JD, Yan J, Zacks DN, Jayasundera KT. Worldwide Argus II implantation: recommendations to optimize patient outcomes. BMC Ophthalmol. 2016;16(1):52. https://doi.org/10.1186/s12886-016-0225-1.

Hayes JS, Yin VT, Piyathaisere D, Weiland JD, Humayun MS, Dagnelie G. Visually guided performance of simple tasks using simulated prosthetic vision. Artif Organs. 2003;27(11):1016–28.

Held R, Hein AV. Adaptation of disarranged hand-eye coordination contingent upon re-afferent stimulation. Percept Mot Skills. 1958;8:87–90.

Ho AC, Humayun MS, Dorn JD, da Cruz L, Dagnelie G, Handa J, Barale PO, Sahel JA, Stanga PE, Hafezi F, Safran AB, Salzmann J, Santos A, Birch D, Spencer R, Cideciyan AV, de Juan E, Duncan JL, Eliott D, Fawzi A, Olmos de Koo LC, Brown GC, Haller JA, Regillo CD, Del Priore LV, Arditi A, Geruschat DR, Greenberg RJ. Long-term results from an epiretinal prosthesis to restore sight to the blind. Ophthalmology. 2015b;122(8):1547–54. https://doi.org/10.1016/j.ophtha.2015.04.032.

Humayun MS, Dorn JD, da Cruz L, Dagnelie G, Sahel JA, Stanga PE, Cideciyan AV, Duncan JL, Eliott D, Filley E, Ho AC, Santos A, Safran AB, Arditi A, Del Priore LV, Greenberg RJ. Interim results from the international trial of Second Sight's visual prosthesis. Ophthalmology. 2012;119(4):779–88. https://doi.org/10.1016/j.ophtha.2011.09.028.

Jeter PE, Rozanski C, Massof RW, Adeyemo O, Dagnelie G, PLoVR Study Group. Development of the ultra low vision-visual functioning questionnaire (ULV-VFQ) as part of the prosthetic low vision rehabilitation (PLoVR) curriculum. Transl Vis Sci Technol. 2017;6(3):11.

Jones BW, Marc RE. Retinal remodeling during retinal degeneration. Exp Eye Res. 2005;81(2):123–37.

Kelley AJ, Yang L, Dagnelie G. The effects of stabilization, font scaling and practice on reading in simulated prosthetic vision. Invest Ophthalmol Vis Sci. 2004;45(ARVO Ann Mtg):E-abstr #5436.

Legge GE, Ross JA, Luebker A, LaMay JM. Psychophysics of reading. VIII. The Minnesota low-vision reading test. Optom Vis Sci. 1989;66(12):843–53.

Mahadevappa M, Weiland JD, Yanai D, Fine I, Greenberg RJ, Humayun MS. Perceptual thresholds and electrode impedance in three retinal prosthesis subjects. IEEE Trans Neural Syst Rehabil Eng. 2005;13(2):201–6.

Massof R, Rubin G. Visual function assessment questionnaires. Surv Ophthalmol. 2001;45(6):531–48.

Massof RW, Ahmadian L, Grover LL, Deremeik JT, Goldstein JE, Rainey C, Epstein C, Barnett GD. The activity inventory: an adaptive visual function questionnaire. Optom Vis Sci. 2007;84(8):763–74.

Mueller V, Wang L, Ostrin LA, Barnett GD, Dagnelie G. Meander mazes: eye-hand coordination in simulated prosthetic vision. Invest Ophthalmol Vis Sci. 2007;48:ARVO E-abstr #2548.

Rizzo JF 3rd, Wyatt J, Loewenstein J, Kelly S, Shire D. Perceptual efficacy of electrical stimulation of human retina with a microelectrode array during short-term surgical trials. Invest Ophthalmol Vis Sci. 2003;44(12):5362–9.

Roessler G, Laube T, Brockmann C, Kirschkamp T, Mazinani B, Goertz M, Koch C, Krisch I, Sellhaus B, Trieu HK, Weis J, Bornfeld N, Rothgen H, Messner A, Mokwa W, Walter P. Implantation and explantation of a wireless epiretinal retina implant device: observations during the EPIRET3 prospective clinical trial. Invest Ophthalmol Vis Sci. 2009;50(6):3003–8.

Sabbah N, Authie CN, Sanda N, Mohand-Said S, Sahel JA, Safran AB. Importance of eye position on spatial localization in blind subjects wearing an Argus II retinal prosthesis. Invest Ophthalmol Vis Sci. 2014;55(12):8259–66. https://doi.org/10.1167/iovs.14-15392.

Stronks HC, Dagnelie G. The functional performance of the Argus II retinal prosthesis. Expert Rev Med Devices. 2014;11(1):23–30. https://doi.org/10.1586/17434440.2014.862494.

Thompson RW, Barnett GD, Humayun MS, Dagnelie G. Facial recognition using simulated prosthetic pixelized vision. Invest Ophthalmol Vis Sci. 2003;44(11):5035–42.

Wang L, Yang L, Dagnelie G. Virtual wayfinding using simulated prosthetic vision in gaze-locked viewing. Optom Vis Sci. 2008;85(11):E1057–63.

Zrenner E. Fighting blindness with microelectronics. Sci Transl Med. 2013;5(210):210ps216. https://doi.org/10.1126/scitranslmed.3007399.

Zrenner E, Bartz-Schmidt KU, Benav H, Besch D, Bruckmann A, Gabel VP, Gekeler F, Greppmaier U, Harscher A, Kibbel S, Koch J, Kusnyerik A, Peters T, Stingl K, Sachs H, Stett A, Szurman P, Wilhelm B, Wilke R. Subretinal electronic chips allow blind patients to read letters and combine them to words. Proc Biol Sci. 2011;278(1711):1489–97. https://doi.org/10.1098/rspb.2010.1747.

Chapter 7
Retinal Prostheses: Other Therapies and Future Directions

Olivier Goureau, Christelle Monville, Antoine Chaffiol, Gregory Gauvain, Serge Picaud, Jens Duebel, and José-Alain Sahel

Introduction

Retinitis pigmentosa (RP), related inherited retinal dystrophies, and age-related retinal degenerative diseases are major courses of yet incurable visual impairment and blindness due to final loss of photoreceptor cells. Depending on the pathology, the type of degenerated cells, and the stage of the disease, several major therapeutic approaches suited to one or more disease stages have been described (reviewed in Jacobson and Cideciyan 2010). These include gene therapy (gene replacement or gene supplementation) to correct the disease-causing genetic defect and associated biochemical abnormalities, neuroprotection (trophic factors) to prevent or slow down the progressive degeneration of

O. Goureau, Ph.D. (✉) • A. Chaffiol, Ph.D. • G. Gauvain, Ph.D. • S. Picaud, Ph.D.
J. Duebel, Ph.D. (✉)
Institut de la Vision, Sorbonne Universités, UPMC Univ Paris 6, INSERM UMRS_968, CNRS UMR 7210, Paris, France
e-mail: olivier.goureau@inserm.fr; antoine.chaffiol@inserm.fr; gregory.gauvain@inserm.fr; serge.picaud@inserm.fr; jens.duebel@inserm.fr

C. Monville, Ph.D.
Université Evry Val Essonne, ISTEM, Paris, France
e-mail: cmonville@istem.fr

J.-A. Sahel, M.D.
Institut de la Vision, Sorbonne Universités, UPMC Univ Paris 6, INSERM UMRS_968, CNRS UMR 7210, Paris, France

Centre Hospitalier National d'Ophtalmologie des Quinze-Vingts, DHU Sight Restore, INSERM-DHOS CIC, Paris, France

Fondation Ophtalmologique Adolphe de Rothschild, Paris, France

Department of Ophthalmology, The University of Pittsburgh School of Medicine, Pittsburgh, PA 15213, USA
e-mail: j.sahel@gmail.com

© Springer International Publishing AG 2018
M.S. Humayun, L.C. Olmos de Koo (eds.), *Retinal Prosthesis*, Essentials in Ophthalmology, https://doi.org/10.1007/978-3-319-67260-1_7

photoreceptors, retinal prostheses to stimulate the visual system and substitute for the usual input from photoreceptors, and cell transplantation. Gene therapy appears a suitable therapeutic approach in the early stages of retinal degeneration in which the photoreceptor density and morphology and, specifically, the cone outer segments are (partially) preserved. Cell therapy by replacing degenerated retinal pigmented epithelium (RPE) is a very promising approach to prevent photoreceptor loss in specific retinal diseases. For the most advanced stages of the disease in which the inner nuclear neurons and circuitry remain relatively preserved for extended periods of time after the photoreceptor loss, retinal prosthesis, optogenetics, and cell therapy by photoreceptor replacement provide alternative approaches for vision restoration.

Optogenetic Therapy

The success of clinical trials on retinal prostheses demonstrated that the electrical stimulation of retinal neurons from blind patients can induce visual perception. The optogenetic approach is an alternative therapeutic strategy, which is currently being evaluated in rodents and nonhuman primates, and should soon enter into clinical trials. The idea of optogenetics is to convert light-insensitive retinal neurons into "artificial photoreceptors" by using light-sensitive opsins, such as microbial opsins, which are derived from bacteria, algae, or other sources. These optogenetic tools can be targeted to specific cell types of the retina with viral vectors. Like an electrical implant, an optogenetic approach works independently of the genetic cause of the disease. Thus, optogenetic-based gene therapy should be applicable to a broad range of patients with rare genetic diseases, such as RP, as well as to more common diseases, such as age-related macular degeneration (AMD), by introducing a gene into the residual retinal neurons using adeno-associated viral vectors (AAVs). An advantage of the optogenetic approach is that injecting a viral vector into the eye does not require a complicated surgery. Another major benefit of optogenetics is the control of neural activity at high spatial resolution which has the potential to restore vision at high acuity levels. Recent gene therapy trials showed successful results in the treatment of Leber congenital amaurosis (Bainbridge et al. 2008; Cideciyan et al. 2009; Maguire et al. 2008; Simonelli et al. 2010) or choroideremia (MacLaren et al. 2014), and promising results were obtained after reinjection of previously treated patients in the contralateral eye (Bennett et al. 2012). These studies have demonstrated the safety and feasibility of gene therapy in the human eye by focusing on the replacement of specific genes, and they pave the way for novel strategies that are mutation independent, such as optogenetic approaches. This chapter describes the various forms of optogenetic therapy strategies using microbial opsins, but it also addresses other approaches based on vertebrate opsins or photosensitizing pharmacological agents.

Cell Type-Specific Targeting of Microbial Opsins: Patient-Tailored Optogenetic Approaches

In retinal degenerative diseases, such as RP or AMD, photoreceptors are affected by degeneration. In RP, rod photoreceptors degenerate first, followed by the progressive loss of cone outer segments, leaving the outer retina with remaining "dormant" cones, i.e., cones lacking their photosensitive part but still alive. At later stages, these surviving cones can disappear as well, while bipolar, horizontal, and amacrine cells remain present. The remnant retinal circuitry is then deeply modified compared to a healthy retina (Krishnamoorthy et al. 2016; Marc et al. 2014). Therefore, depending on the stage of degeneration of the retina, different optogenetic therapies seem to be available for the patient: in the early stage of the disease, activity could be restored in cones lacking their outer segments. When cones are degenerated, one could generate artificial photoreceptors from the inner nuclear layer (INL) cells, such as bipolar cells or amacrine cells. Finally, in late stages of the disease, once bipolar cells are no longer present, retinal ganglion cells (RGCs) could be targeted (Fig. 7.1).

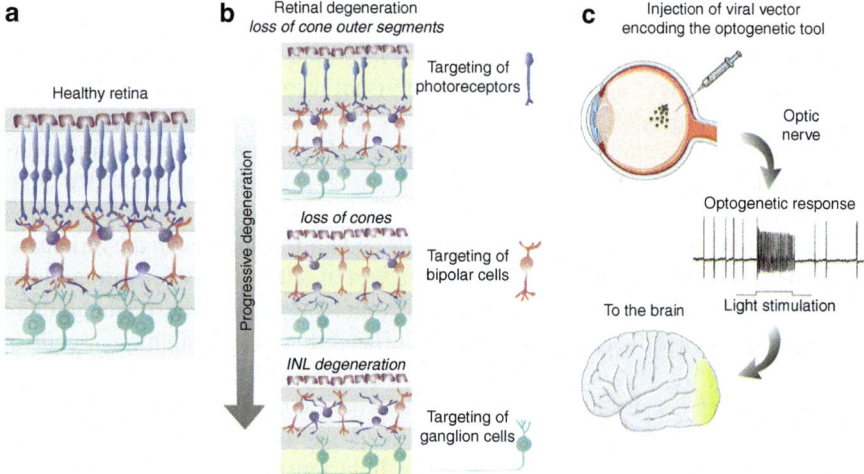

Fig. 7.1 Cell type-specific optogenetic vision restoration strategies are dependent on the stage of retinal degeneration. (**a**) Healthy retina. (**b**) Retinal degeneration stages and corresponding optogenetic strategies. At early stages rod photoreceptor degeneration is followed by cone outer segments loss (*top*); later cone cell bodies also degenerate (*center*). At late stages of the disease, important circuitry remodeling occurs in the inner nuclear layer (INL, *bottom*). Retinal pigment epithelium cells are shown in *brown*, photoreceptors in *blue*, horizontal and amacrine cells in *purple*, bipolar cells in *red*, and retinal ganglion cells in *green*. (**c**) After an intravitreal injection of the engineered viral vector coding for the optogenetic tool into the patient's eye, transfected retinal cells can respond to light. The example trace shows a light response from a mouse retinal ganglion cell expressing ChR2. The global signal output originating from the treated retina is then transmitted via the optic nerve to the brain

The first study that used an optogenetic approach to reactivate the retina of blind mice was performed in rd1 mice, a model of photoreceptor degeneration. This pioneering work showed that expression of channelrhodopsin-2 (ChR2) in RGCs can confer light sensitivity to a previously blind retina (Bi et al. 2006), which was followed by other studies (Tomita et al. 2007, 2009, 2010; Zhang et al. 2009; Greenberg et al. 2011). In order to evaluate the potential of clinical translation, ChR2 has been expressed with an AAV in the marmoset, a nonhuman primate (Ivanova et al. 2010). This work demonstrated that RGCs of the marmoset retina can indeed be activated by ChR2. However, the eye of marmoset is much smaller than the human eye; thus, the efficacy of viral vectors (AAV) to express microbial opsins has to be further evaluated in species that are phylogenetically closer to humans, such as macaques. Targeting of RGCs could be a therapeutic strategy for blind patients who show advanced degeneration of the INL; but it is important to note that targeting of RGCs with ChR2 would lead to an ON response in all RGCs, i.e., all cells would be turned into ON-type cells. Moreover, the image processing capability of inner retinal circuits cannot be utilized with this approach. On the other hand, clinical studies with epi-retinal implants have demonstrated that the human cortex has the capability to make use from a visual code that is triggered by direct stimulation of RGCs.

Targeting of ChR-2 to retinal ON bipolar cells is an alternative approach that offers the benefit that neural circuits upstream of RGCs are utilized. A pioneering study has shown that targeting ON bipolar cells with a specific promoter via electroporation (Lagali et al. 2008) can restore visual responses on the retinal, cortical, and behavioral level of treated blind mice. In a next step, electroporation was replaced by viral gene delivery that is suitable for future clinical applications (Doroudchi et al. 2011). More recently, by using viral vectors especially engineered for retinal infection (Dalkara et al. 2013), it has been demonstrated that the activation of ON bipolar cells can induce ON and OFF responses in the retina and in the visual cortex (Cronin et al. 2014; Mace et al. 2015). This activation of the ON/OFF pathway is mediated by the inner retinal circuitry. Unfortunately, there is currently no viral vector specifically and efficiently transducing bipolar cells in primates.

The discovery of residual photoreceptors in mouse models of retinal degeneration, as well as in blind patients, suggested the possibility to reactivate these "dormant" photoreceptors that have lost their light-sensitive outer segments. The expression of the light-sensitive chloride pump, halorhodopsin, showed that it is possible to reactivate these "dormant" cones in blind mice. Surprisingly, complex visual functions, such as center-surround antagonism or direction selectivity, were restored in these treated retinas (Busskamp et al. 2010). By using cultured postmortem human retina (Fradot et al. 2011), researchers were able to show that halorhodopsin could also be expressed in human photoreceptors and be functional (Busskamp et al. 2010). Screening with optical coherence tomography (OCT) confirmed the presence of such "dormant" photoreceptors in blind RP patients (Busskamp et al. 2010). Those patients could be eligible candidates for future clinical trials. However, current in vivo tests in nonhuman primate did not yet reach sufficient level of halorhodopsin expression (unpublished data). Therefore, in the present state of our knowledge, and taking into account diverse retinal remodeling (Marc et al. 2014; Jones et al. 2016), targeting RGCs seems to be the first approach to move into clinical trials (Fig. 7.1c).

The Choice of the Optogenetic Tool

As we have described above, the success of optogenetic strategies depends on the specific targeting of a population of surviving retinal neurons by using tailored viral vectors. The efficacy of this vector will be determined by (1) the viral capsid and (2) the promoter, controlling the transgene expression; but the expressed element of the vector will be the optogenetic tool. The choice of the optogenetic tool is critical to the success of the therapy. The majority of the published studies using optogenetic tools to restore vision used the microbial opsin ChR2 (Bi et al. 2006; Tomita et al. 2007, 2010; Lagali et al. 2008; Ivanova and Pan 2009; Zhang et al. 2009; Ivanova et al. 2010; Doroudchi et al. 2011; Mace et al. 2015). In order to translate the encouraging proofs of concept obtained in these studies to the clinic, careful tailoring of the opto-genes is needed. Two different paths are currently explored; one is based on the identification or engineering of microbial opsins with improved biophysical properties, and the other path is to use vertebrate opsins or proteins engineered from vertebrate opsins.

Microbial Opsins

Microbial opsins are retinal-binding proteins that capture light energy and use it to either actively pump ions across cell membrane or to open channels allowing a passive flow of ions across cell membrane. When introduced into non-light-sensitive cells, microbial opsins enable to control their activity by using light as a stimulus. The first steps in the discovery of microbial opsins were made in the 1970s by Oesterhelt and Stoeckenius, when they identified bacteriorhodopsin, a rhodopsin-like protein from the purple membrane of *Halobacterium halobium* that pumps protons under illumination (Oesterhelt and Stoeckenius 1971), followed by the discovery of halorhodopsin, a light-driven hyperpolarizing chloride pump from Archaebacteria (Matsuno-Yagi and Mukohata 1977). A major breakthrough was then the discovery of channelrhodopsin, a blue light-sensitive cation channel from the green algae *Chlamydomonas reinhardtii* (Nagel et al. 2002, 2003), followed by the demonstration that, upon introduction of a microbial opsin, neurons became responsive to light (Boyden et al. 2005).

The optogenetic toolbox was later expanded by the identification of multiple opsins able to activate or to silence neuronal activity (Chow et al. 2010; Cosentino et al. 2015; Hausser 2014). Since then, different variants have been discovered with increased light sensitivity (Kleinlogel et al. 2011; Pan et al.

2014) in order to increase the efficacy of vision restoration strategies. Indeed, they reduce the amount of required membrane-bound opsins needed for optogenetic stimulation. This is in particular the case of the "CatCh" protein that shows an increased light sensitivity based on its permeability to calcium ions. However, despite these improvements, the light intensity required for the stimulation of microbial opsins is still very high, compared to the intrinsic opsins from a human eye. A major bottleneck of channelrhodopsin-based vision restoration strategies is that stimulation with blue light is needed, having the high risk of inducing photochemical damage in the retina, as well as in the RPE (Ham et al. 1978; Rozanowska et al. 1995; Wu et al. 2006; Organisciak and Vaughan 2010). Since the damage potential of red light is vastly lower than that of blue light, there has been great interest in the development of red-shifted channelrhodopsin variants, such as ReaChR or Chrimson (Lin et al. 2013; Klapoetke et al. 2014). These novel opsins provide a therapeutic approach that can safely work in the human eye by using red-shifted stimulation. Finally, the risk of immune responses in human retina to microbial opsins is an important unknown, and the tolerability of microbial opsins has to be evaluated carefully in the nonhuman primate retina, before moving to clinical trials.

Other Optogenetic Tools

An interesting alternative for optogenetic applications are vertebrate opsins, such as rhodopsin or melanopsin. Compared to microbial opsins, the light sensitivity of vertebrate opsins is much higher, since the photon-triggered signals are amplified by G-protein-coupled signaling cascades. It has been demonstrated that the expression of melanopsin in blind mice can lead to light-induced responses at low light levels (Lin et al. 2008). However, the slow kinetics of melanopsin does not allow for light stimulation at sufficient temporal resolution. In a recent study, a melanopsin-mGluR6 chimera expressed in bipolar cells showed that the temporal property of melanopsin has been improved toward faster kinetics (van Wyk et al. 2015). The expression of rhodopsin in bipolar cells demonstrated that light responses can be elicited even at indoor light levels (Gaub et al. 2015; Cehajic-Kapetanovic et al. 2015). However, bleaching of rhodopsin remains an important challenge, because for the chromophore recycling (Strauss, 2005) close interaction of the retina with the RPE is needed, which could be a problem in many retinal degenerative diseases.

Finally, a photochemical approach has also been proposed to resensitize the retina of blind patients. The idea is based on ocular injection of chemical photoswitches that can trigger the opening of ion channels upon light stimulation. This approach has now been validated in the retina ex vivo and in vivo for blind rodents (Polosukhina et al. 2012; Tochitsky et al. 2014). A major drawback for therapy is that it requires injections of photosensitizing molecules in the eye at regular time intervals. The need of repeated injections is a clear bottleneck, but this approach has the advantage to be reversible in case of major side effects.

Future Perspectives

The optogenetic approach allows us to confer light sensitivity to specific cell types in the retina by using AAVs, which have already been used as a safe gene delivery tool in clinical studies. Viral vectors, especially designed for ocular gene delivery, in combination with novel optogenetic tools provide us with new therapeutic perspectives for a wide range of inherited retinal degenerative diseases, such as RP, as well as common age-related eye diseases, such as AMD. A key advantage of optogenetics is that it allows control of neural activity at high spatial resolution. Thus, an optogenetic therapy could enable to restore vision at high acuity levels.

Cell Therapy

State of the Art

Cell replacement therapies have been historically viewed as a potential vision restoration strategy for retinal degenerative diseases with significant cell damage. These therapeutics aim at replacing the lost retinal cells using stem cells, progenitor cells, and mature neural retinal cells. One of the main advantages of cell therapies is that they are mutation-independent and can be used in a wide range of retinal degeneration conditions.

The eye represents an ideal target for cell therapies as (1) it is easily accessible and small (low number of cells would be sufficient for therapy), (2) it is highly compartmentalized (permitting to target different ocular tissues such as vitreous or subretinal space), and (3) the eye is a prototypic immune-privileged tissue that resists immunogenic inflammation through multiple mechanisms (Streilein et al. 2002; Forrester 2009). Moreover, the development of noninvasive imaging approaches, such as optical coherence tomography and adaptive optics, is of great value in both diagnosis and follow-up after transplantation. Finally, the contralateral eye can serve as an internal control in evaluation outcomes.

Patients suffering from retinal degeneration typically lose RPE cells, photoreceptors, or both. Therefore, two main cell sources can be considered: (1) RPE cells to replace dysfunctional or degenerated RPE and to prevent photoreceptor cell loss and (2) photoreceptor precursors to repair the degenerating neural retina. In this context, human pluripotent stem cells (hPSCs) are an attractive alternative to ocular-derived stem cell populations as a potentially inexhaustible source of donor cells. They can be maintained indefinitely in an undifferentiated state in vitro and demonstrate the capacity to differentiate into cells from all three germ layers (endoderm, mesoderm, and ectoderm). This part of the review focuses on encouraging results in animal models of retinal degeneration after transplantation of RPE cells and photoreceptors derived from hPSCs, and on stem cell-based therapies targeting RP and AMD currently under clinical evaluation.

Cell Transplantation Using hPSCs

Human embryonic stem cells (hESCs) have been the best studied since their first isolation from the inner cell mass of a blastocyst (Thomson et al. 1998). The discovery in 2007 by the group of S. Yamanaka that somatic cells can be reprogrammed with four specific transcription factors (POU5F1, SOX2, KLF4, and c-MYC) into an ES cell-like pluripotent state, known as human-induced pluripotent stem cells (hiPSCs) (Takahashi et al. 2007), offers a new promising source of cells for transplantation approaches, especially in an autologous context.

Based on the identification of the specific molecular signals required for neuroectodermal identity adoption, eye field specification, and retinal differentiation, the guided differentiation of mouse ES cells and also of hESCs and hiPSCs toward retinal lineages has progressed rapidly in the last decade (reviews in Song and Bharti 2016; Leach and Clegg 2015; Wiley et al. 2015; Nazari et al. 2015; Borooah et al. 2013).

RPE Cell Replacement: RPE Cells vs. RPE Sheets

The RPE provides essential support for the long-term preservation of retinal integrity and visual function (Strauss, 2005). For instance, RPE cells (1) control nutrient and metabolite flow to and from the retina, replenish 11-*cis* retinal by reisomerizing all-*trans* retinal generated during photoconversion, (2) phagocyte daily a portion of the outer segments of photoreceptors, and (3) secrete cytokines that locally control the innate and adaptive immune systems (Strauss, 2005). It is also part of the blood-retina barrier and, together with the selectively permeable Bruch's membrane, provides control over ion, nutrient, and metabolite transport between the retina and the fenestrated capillaries of the choroid. Given the intimate anatomical and functional relationship of RPE cells and photoreceptors, it is not surprising that any disease or abnormality that affects the RPE displays problems with vision.

The treatment of RPE-associated degenerative eye diseases by cell therapy was first proposed by Gouras and collaborators in the early 1980s (Gouras et al. 1984, 1985). This group successfully transplanted RPE cells in a monkey model, demonstrating the feasibility of such approach. By the end of the 1980s, it was well established that RPE cells can not only be transplanted in degenerated retina but also can delay photoreceptor degeneration in a rat model of retinal degeneration (Lopez et al. 1989), opening the path to the development of therapeutic cell-based strategies. Laboratories from all over the world developed and tested methods to produce cells that can replace defective or degenerated endogenous RPE cells. Several cell sources have been evoked for RPE cell therapy rising from the adult eye, autologous RPE cells harvested from the peripheral retina (Wang et al. 2008) and allogenic RPE graft harvested from cadavers, and recently a new potential source has been identified with the discovery of human RPE stem cells (Salero et al. 2012).

Significant research efforts have focused on finding the ideal methods for efficiently deriving RPE cells from hPSCs. It has been well demonstrated that hPSCs have the capacity to "spontaneously" differentiate to RPE cells using the continuous adherent culture method and the embryoid body method (reviewed in Leach and Clegg 2015), but the efficiency could be low and lead to multiple cell doublings to obtain the sufficient number of cells for transplantation. In parallel, protocols that use knowledge of the developmental biology of the eye have been successfully developed (Song and Bharti 2016). Many research labs have now optimized direct RPE differentiation protocols using growth factors and small molecules (Leach and Clegg 2015). hPSCs are first engaged to express neuroectodermal characteristics by their exposition to inhibitors of the WNT signaling pathway (DKK1/NODAL and LEFTY-A). Then neuroectodermal progenitor cells are differentiated into RPE cells using a culture medium that does not contain fibroblast growth factor 2 (FGF2) and in the presence of activin A. The combination of chetomin, an inhibitor of hypoxia-inducible factors, with nicotinamide yielded a highly pure hPSC-derived RPE cell population that displayed many of the morphological, molecular, and functional characteristics of native RPE (Maruotti et al. 2015).

The most innovating approaches are represented by the generation of tridimensional retinal structures, corresponding to optic cup-, optic vesicle-like structures and more mature retinal organoids. These protocols were used to simultaneously generate RPE cells from hESCs and hiPSCs in a reproducible manner (Meyer et al. 2011; Nakano et al. 2012; Zhong et al. 2014; Reichman et al. 2014).

Significant research efforts are focusing on finding the ideal method for transplanting hPSC-derived RPE cells into the subretinal space. Optimizing RPE transplantation procedures resulted in the development of two different therapeutic strategies: (1) introducing a cell suspension of RPE cells into the subretinal space and allowing the donor cells to integrate within the host retina and (2) transplanting polarized sheets of RPE cells to allow for improved safety and better clinical outcomes, since normal RPE functions are dependent on specific cellular features of its apical and basal domains (Buchholz et al. 2009; Nazari et al. 2015).

Regarding efficacy, most preclinical animal data suggest that cells injected in the subretinal space as a suspension often fail to survive at long term compared to polarized RPE monolayer (Carr et al. 2009; Diniz et al. 2013). Indeed, transplanted RPE cells were almost not detectable 13 weeks posttransplantation in two studies performed in Royal College of Surgeons (RCS) rats and nude rodents (Carr et al. 2009; Diniz et al. 2013), while only 0.2% of RPE cells were still present 28 weeks postinjection in another study (Wang et al. 2005). In addition, the viability and ability for RPE cells to regain a fully differentiated phenotype in the subretinal space were even lower when the integrity of the underlying substrate, the Bruch's membrane, was disturbed (Booij et al. 2010). Finally, the injection of a cell suspension could only produce a transient functional recovery due to the death of RPE cells that do not benefit from the foundation of a basement membrane ensuring their correct polarization, between 10 and 15 weeks after injection (Carr et al. 2009). Altogether these results suggest that permanent implantation of a polarized RPE monolayer that exhibits the physiology of its natural counterpart represents a favorable alternative to RPE cell suspension (Stanzel et al. 2014). For that purpose, multiple different substrates have been tried for generating a polarized RPE monolayer on a scaffold (Jha and Bharti 2015). Among those, non-biodegradable synthetic scaffolds like polyester or parylene substrates have been tested and developed for clinical applications (Hu et al. 2012; Ramsden et al. 2013; Lu et al. 2014; Stanzel et al. 2014), and poly-lactic-co-glycolic acid (PLGA) is under development (Liu et al. 2014; Song and Bharti 2016). Several parameters must be taken into consideration, such as thickness, mechanical properties, and biodegradation, to prevent additional damage of the retina and improve the interactions between the retina and RPE (Kador and Goldberg 2012). We are currently optimizing a cell therapy with allogeneic hESC-derived RPE cells over a biological substrate that consists of polarized hESC-derived RPE cells cultured on human amniotic membrane. This membrane commonly used in ocular surface reconstruction (He et al. 2014) presents significant advantages such as anti-inflammatory and antimicrobial properties (Niknejad et al. 2008). The group of M. Takahashi developed a strategy based on RPE sheets transplantation without any matrix or scaffold using an ingenious system (Kamao et al. 2014). hiPSC-derived RPE were cultured onto Transwell inserts coated with collagen. When the RPE cells reach confluency and form a typical cobblestone pigmented epithelium, the RPE sheet is removed from the insert by a collagenase treatment and the size of the RPE sheet is then adjusted using a laser microdissection system (Kamao et al. 2014).

Ongoing and future clinical trials will show whether the transplantation of RPE tissue (with or without artificial scaffold biodegradable or not) will provide better survival and integration (thus better functional outcome) than the injection of RPE cell suspension.

PR Cell Replacement: Precursors of PR and Retinal Sheets

Protocols guiding hPSC differentiation have been developed during the last decade by trying to mimic the successive developmental steps in vitro: neural induction and eye field and retinal specification, with the commitment and the differentiation of retinal progenitor cells (RPCs) to specific cell types of the neuroretina (reviewed in Wiley et al. 2015; Nazari et al. 2015; Borooah et al. 2013).

A variety of retinal differentiation protocols combined a serum-free floating culture of embryoid bodies (called SFEB system) and adherent cultures by plating embryoid bodies that are able, in principle, to generate cells of all the three germ layers (endoderm, ectoderm, and mesoderm). These stepwise 3D-2D protocols demonstrated the requirement of preventing the endogenous activation of bone morphogenetic protein (BMP)/transforming growth factor β (TGFβ) and WNT pathways as well as the activation of insulin growth factor I (IGF-1)/INSULIN pathway at early stage of cultures to commit the cells toward a neuroectodermal lineage and secondarily toward a retinal cell fate (Reh et al. 2010). Indeed, these conditions allowed the identification of cells expressing several eye field transcription factors, such as RX, PAX6, LHX2, and SIX3. These RPCs can be differentiated into the photoreceptor lineage by addition, at specific time points on the 2D step, of retinoic acid, Sonic HedgeHog (SHH), taurine, and triiodothyronine (T3) (Wiley et al. 2015; Borooah et al. 2013). Incorporation of an additional 3D step allowed the self-formation of neuroepithelial structures, which corresponded ontogenetically to the optic vesicle (OV) stage (Meyer et al. 2011; Phillips et al. 2012). Following isolation, floating OV-like structures continued to differentiate toward the photoreceptor lineage, with the expression of mature photoreceptor markers such as RHODOPSIN or S-OPSIN around 100 days in culture (Meyer et al. 2011). Recently, improvement of this stepwise 3D/2D/3D (SFEB floating/plating/isolated OV-like structures in suspension) protocol of differentiation demonstrated that hiPSCs could efficiently generate retinal structures that were properly laminated with the presence of mature photoreceptors forming outer segment disks (Zhong et al. 2014).

Over the last few years, interesting papers from the Sasai's group based on their previous study using mouse ES cells (Eiraku et al. 2011) reported the formation of a bilayered optic cup using re-aggregated hESCs cultured as SFEB in the presence of Matrigel and WNT inhibitor and SHH agonist in very specific time windows (Nakano et al. 2012). These culture conditions allowed the identification of photoreceptors within neural rosettes formed in the 3D structures by expression of CRX, RECOVERIN, and RHODOPSIN from day 35 to day 120 (Nakano et al. 2012). Successive steps of BMP4 priming followed by addition of FGF receptor inhibitor, Glycogen synthase kinase-3 (GSK3) inhibitor, and, finally, retinoic acid and taurine addition permitted the self-formation of well-laminated neural retina without modifying the rate and the yield of photoreceptor generation (Kuwahara et al. 2015).

Moving toward future clinical applications requires the development of simple and reliable retinal differentiation process, which also should reduce the need for exogenous factors (Matrigel, serum, etc.). In this context, Reichman et al. recently developed a GMP-compatible protocol starting from overgrowing adherent hiPSCs in pro-neural medium that allowed simultaneous generation of RPE cells and self-forming retinal organoids comprising photoreceptors (Reichman et al. 2014).

Historically, the first attempts of retinal neuron replacement using cells derived from pluripotent stem cells concerned the intravitreally or subretinally injections of neural progenitors derived from human ES cells into immune-suppressed rats (Banin et al. 2006). Very low percentage of the engrafted neural progenitors (<1.5%) expressed photoreceptor markers indicating an insufficient competence for photoreceptor generation. Nevertheless, any tumor formation was detected by 16 weeks post-operation (Banin et al. 2006). Recent papers confirmed that both hESC- and hiPSC-derived neural progenitors remained as phenotypically uncommitted progenitors following transplantation but they are effective in preserving vision in blind animal models (Lu et al. 2013; Tsai et al. 2015).

To date, there are very few studies using hESC- or hiPSC-derived retinal cells to replace photoreceptors. A larger number of studies have been subsequently conducted by using differentiated mouse PSCs as source of cells for transplantation (Tucker et al. 2011; West et al. 2012; Garita-Hernandez et al. 2013; Gonzalez-Cordero et al. 2013; Decembrini et al. 2014). Interestingly photoreceptor precursors derived from 3D mouse ESC cultures were capable to integrate into adult host retina and to mature into new photoreceptors, without any tumor formation (Gonzalez-Cordero et al. 2013; Decembrini et al. 2014). Unfortunately, no assessment of visual function has been performed in rodent model of blindness due to the low number of integrated cells (<0.3%). Nevertheless, histological analysis of integrated mouse ES cell-derived rods demonstrated that newly formed photoreceptors were able to connect with the existing circuitry in retina of blind mice (Gonzalez-Cordero et al. 2013). In the case of large animals, it has been reported that rhodopsin-positive photoreceptors derived from swine iPS cells can integrate into the damaged retina of swine (Zhou et al. 2011).

The group of T. Reh was the first to report transplantation of hPSCs directed to a retinal fate (Lamba et al. 2009, 2010). According to their "SFEB retinal differentiation" protocol (Reh et al. 2010), hESCs were differentiated for 3 weeks, and between 50,000 and 80,000 "retinal cells" were transplanted into the subretinal space of adult wild-type mice without any prior selection. Some transplanted cells were found after 6 weeks to be integrated in the retina and showed expression of rod and cone photoreceptor markers (Lamba et al. 2009). A similar result has been obtained with the transplantation of retinal cells derived from hiPSCs into the subretinal space of adult wild-type mice (Lamba et al. 2010). In order to determine whether these integrated photoreceptors were functional, they performed transplantation experiments into blind mice, where none ERG response could be recorded. 2–3 weeks after subretinal injection of hESC-derived retinal cells, a partial restoration of light response was detected by ERG analysis, where the amplitude of the B-wave response was correlated with the number of integrated cells (Lamba et al. 2009).

In the case of very severe degenerations and loss of outer nuclear layer (ONL), transplantation of retinal tissue rather than dissociated photoreceptor cells could be required. The development of recent innovative protocols allowing the generation of retinal organoids from hPSCs (Meyer et al. 2011; Nakano et al. 2012; Zhong et al. 2014; Reichman et al. 2014), will be very useful to derived transplantable retinal tissues. The group of M. Takahashi has already performed the proof of concept with the transplantation of mouse ES-derived retinal sheets containing a defined ONL into a ONL-depleted host retina in *rd1* mice (Assawachananont et al. 2014). Recently the same group reported a similar approach with hESC-derived retinal tissue in a new primate model of retinal degeneration (Shirai et al. 2016). Even though few animals (*n* = 2) have been transplanted, this study showed the maturation of transplanted hESC-derived retinal sheets with the possible integration of grafted photoreceptors with host bipolar cells. Ongoing transplantation studies in animal models will show whether the transplantation of purified photoreceptors or whole retinal tissue is the most adapted for integration and connection of the transplanted cells and less immunogenic.

Trials with Stem Cells

To date, at least 15 ongoing clinical trials are registered at the International Clinical Trials Registry Platform (ICTRP) of the World Health Organization to test stem cell-based replacement therapies for treatment of retinal dystrophies (Dalkara et al. 2016; Klassen 2016). Many types of stem cells were used: retinal derivatives from hPSCs or from fetal tissue, neural stem cells (NSCs), and non-neural stem cells such as mesenchymal stem cells (MSCs) and bone marrow-derived stem cells (BMSCs). Paracrine effects such as anti-apoptotic could explain how NSCs, MSCs, and BMSCs contribute to prolonged retinal cell survival, rather than their ability to generate new retinal cells. In this paragraph, we will focus on stem cell-based therapies using retinal derivatives (Table 7.1).

The first clinical trial has been conducted by Ocata Therapeutics, Inc. (MA, USA) to evaluate the safety and tolerability of a subretinal injection of hESC-derived RPE cells in patients with dry AMD and Stargardt (STGD) (Schwartz et al. 2012, 2015). Increasing doses of cells in suspension have been administered to one eye of nine patients with dry AMD and nine STGD patients (three patients

Table 7.1 Clinical trials based on human retinal cells (initiated or completed as of March 2016)

Sponsor (locations)	Identifiers	Phase	Retinal cell derivatives (cell source)	Target disease
Ocata Therapeutics (USA, UK)	NCT01345006/ NCT02445612	I/II	RPE cells (ES cells)	Stargardt's disease
Ocata Therapeutics (USA, UK)	NCT01344993/ NCT02463344/ NCT02563782	I/II and II	RPE cells (ES cells)	Dry AMD
Ocata Therapeutics (USA)	NCT02122159	I/II	RPE cells (ES cells)	Myopic macular degeneration
CHA Biotech Co. (South Korea)	NCT01674829	I/II	RPE cells (ES cells)	Dry AMD and Stargardt's disease
Cell Cure Neurosciences (Israel)	NCT02286089	I/IIa	RPE cells (ES cells)	Dry AMD
Pfizer/University College London (UK)	NCT01691261	I	Sheet of RPE cells on polyester membrane (ES cells)	AMD
RIKEN Institute (Japan)	UMIN000011929	I	Sheet of RPE cells (autologous iPS cells)	Wet AMD
Regenerative Patch Technologies (USA)	NCT02590692	I	Sheet of RPE cells on parylene membrane (ES cells)	Dry AMD and GA
Southwest Hospital Chongqing (China)	ChiCTR-OCB-15006423	I/II	RPE cells (ES cells)	Macular degeneration
jCyte, Inc. (USA)	NCT02320812	I	Retinal progenitor cells (fetal origin)	RP

in each cohort with 50,000, 100,000, or 150,000 cells). Follow-up testing showed that 10 out of 18 treated eyes had substantial improvements in the first year after transplantation. Median follow-up at 22 months suggests no major safety concerns (no signs of hyperproliferation, tumorigenicity, ectopic tissue formation, or apparent rejection). Adverse events were associated with surgery and immunosuppressive treatment but were not considered related to the hESC-derived cells (Schwartz et al. 2015), providing evidence of the medium- to long-term safety and survival of hESC-derived RPE cell injected as a cell suspension in patients with macular degeneration. Same approaches using cell suspensions of hESC-derived RPE cells have started in South Korea (CHA Biotech Co., Ltd.) and in Israel (Cell Cure Neurosciences Ltd.) in patients with dry AMD and STGD. One-year follow-up for four patients in the Korean study confirmed the safety issues of this approach (Song et al. 2015).

In contrast different groups developed a strategy that intends to transplant hESC-derived RPE cells as an already polarized monolayer. The London Project to Cure Blindness (sponsored by Pfizer) will insert a monolayer sheet of RPE cells cultured on polyester membrane in ten patients with wet AMD and rapid recent vision decline. This polyester matrix has been reported to maintain polarized human RPE cells, and the benefit of the subretinal graft of this tissue-engineering product (TEP) has been shown in the rabbit (Stanzel et al. 2014). Similarly, polarized monolayer of hESC-derived RPE cells attached to a nondegradable parylene membrane has been developed by the California Project to Cure Blindness. This scaffold possesses similar permeability properties of a healthy Bruch's membrane, and the proof of concept with this TEP has been reported in RCS rats and in Yucatan pigs (Nazari et al. 2015; Diniz et al. 2013).

As hiPSCs can be obtained directly from the patient, they have the advantage of being autologous and therefore less immunogenic than hESCs for future cell transplantation studies. In this context, the RIKEN Center for developmental biology in Japan has initiated in the end of 2014 the first phase I/II clinical trial assessing the safety and feasibility of the transplantation of autologous hiPSC-derived RPE for AMD treatment. In implant a sheet of RPE differentiated from hiPSCs previously derived from fibroblasts of one patient suffering from exudative form of AMD has been transplanted to this patient, and five other patients were planned. However due to genetic defects found in the cells from the second patient, this first-in-man clinical trial was suspended (Garber 2015). The National Eye Institute (NIH) and Cellular Dynamics International are also developing an autologous strategy using hiPSCs derived from CD34-positive cells. They will use a polarized RPE monolayer derived from these hiPSCs cultured on a biodegradable poly-lactic-co-glycolic acid scaffold (Song and Bharti 2016).

Another type of cell-based therapy for retinal degeneration approaching clinical translation is the use of human RPCs. The California Institute for Regenerative Medicine, with jCyte company, uses human RPCs obtained from fetal retina and previously expanded in culture. They recently started clinical trials to evaluate the safety of intravitreal injection of these human cells in RP patients. The effects of these cells are expected to be neurotrophic even though their ability to differentiate and integrate into the retina cannot be totally excluded.

Future Challenges

Several preclinical and clinical trials using hPSC-derived retinal cells are ongoing, showing that several protocols following Good manufacturing Practice (GMP) proceduress exist (at least for hESCs), and we are entering a very exciting era leading to different treatments for patients.

In most countries and jurisdictions, the use of cellular products for medical therapy is regulated by governmental agencies to ensure the protection of patients and the prudent use of resources so that novel therapies will be the most widely beneficial for the population. Many technical and regulatory breakthroughs in the last few years have made stem cell-based treatment for retinal degeneration more plausible. During the manufacturing process of hPSC-derived retinal cells, several important limiting key points need to be carefully evaluated, safety, purity, and potency of differentiated cells, according to regulatory guidelines (Schwartz et al. 2012, 2015). Regardless of particular cell type, hPSCs carry additional risks due to their pluripotency. These include the ability to acquire mutations when maintained for prolonged periods in culture, to grow and differentiate into inappropriate cellular phenotypes, to form benign teratomas or malignant outgrowths, and to fail to mature.

As compared to spontaneous differentiation, stepwise developmentally guided methods are certainly more efficient and generally quicker. However, for the clinical translation process of retinal cell differentiation protocols, all parameters need to be evaluated with utmost rigor. According to European and US regulatory guidelines, the production of retinal cells requires to be reproducible and to use fully defined xeno-free media. Moreover, the manufacturer should provide a full traceability of their starting materials (culture media, cytokines, and coating substrates) indicating that they are pathogen-free and produced in a sterile environment. All this selection increases the development steps from the first research protocol to the clinical one. This optimization process faces challenges due to the variation of the non-GMP starting material to the GMP one and to the batch to batch variability of the same product. As to date, protocols to derive and differentiate hiPSCs under GMP-compliant conditions will still have to be secured as recent observation of potential tumorigenic mutations in some of the clinical-grade iPSC line for one AMD patient of the Japanese clinical trial raises concerns (Garber 2015).

Even if subretinal space is largely an immune-privileged site, attention should be drawn toward the fact that surgical trauma during cell transplantation compromises the blood-ocular barrier and subjects surrounding cells to an increased level of recognition and reactions. In order to obtain long-term survival and function of the transplanted cells, we might provide some protection against the inflammatory response that could be triggered at the time of surgery by using robust immunosuppressive regimen (Schwartz et al. 2012, 2015) or intravitreal implants of corticosteroid capsules (Ahmad et al. 2012; Tomkins-Netzer et al. 2014). Generation of hPSC-derived retinal cells with known Human Leucocyte Antigen (HLA) genotypes may reduce risks of rejection (Andrews et al. 2015; Taylor et al. 2005). Gourraud and collaborators developed a probabilistic model and demonstrated that using a bank comprising the 100 iPSC lines with the most frequent HLA in each population would leave out only 22% of the European Americans, but 37% of the Asians, 48% of the Hispanics, and 55% of the African Americans (Gourraud et al. 2012). International strategies started now in order to create such banks, which might be useful as a source of allografts in retinal disorders (Andrews et al. 2015). Finally, because diseases caused by retinal malfunction affect at least 30 millions of people worldwide, a figure that will triple with the increase in the aging population in the next 30–40 years (Wong et al. 2014), industrialization and automation of cell production will have to be considered in the future.

Concluding Remarks

Optogenetic approaches and cell therapy opened new possibilities in the treatment of currently incurable retinal degenerative diseases. Ongoing safety and tolerability prospective clinical trials, both in retinal cell therapy (see Table 7.1) and in optogenetic retinal therapy (ClinicalTrials.gov Identifier: NCT02556736), should provide relevant information and allow to overcome last hurdles to the pursuit of these innovative treatments in human.

Compliance with Ethical Requirements *Olivier Goureau, Christelle Monville, Antoine Chaffiol, Gregory Gauvain*, and *Serge Picaud* declare that they have no conflict of interest.

José-Alain Sahel declares:

Consultant: Pixium Vision, GenSight Biologics, Sanofi-Fovea, Gene Signal, Vision Medicines.
Personal financial interest: Pixium Vision, GenSight Biologics, Chronocam, Chronolife.
Funding sources: LabEx LIFESENSES (ANR-10-LABX-65), Banque publique d'Investissement, Foundation Fighting Blindness.

Jens Duebel declares *funding source*: ERC Starting Grant (OptogenRet 309,776).
No human or animal studies were carried out by the authors for this chapter.

References

Ahmad ZM, Hughes BA, Abrams GW, et al. Combined posterior chamber intraocular lens, vitrectomy, Retisert, and pars plana tube in noninfectious uveitis. Arch Ophthalmol. 2012;130:908–13.
Andrews PW, Baker D, Benvinisty N, et al. Points to consider in the development of seed stocks of pluripotent stem cells for clinical applications: international stem cell banking initiative (ISCBI). Regen Med. 2015;10:1–44.
Assawachananont J, Mandai M, Okamoto S, et al. Transplantation of embryonic and induced pluripotent stem cell-derived 3D retinal sheets into retinal degenerative mice. Stem Cell Rep. 2014;2:662–74.

Bainbridge JW, Smith AJ, Barker SS, et al. Effect of gene therapy on visual function in Leber's congenital amaurosis. N Engl J Med. 2008;358:2231–9.

Banin E, Obolensky A, Idelson M, et al. Retinal incorporation and differentiation of neural precursors derived from human embryonic stem cells. Stem Cells. 2006;24:246–57.

Bennett J, Ashtari M, Wellman J, et al. AAV2 gene therapy readministration in three adults with congenital blindness. Sci Transl Med. 2012;4:120ra15.

Bi A, Cui J, Ma YP, et al. Ectopic expression of a microbial-type rhodopsin restores visual responses in mice with photoreceptor degeneration. Neuron. 2006;50:23–33.

Booij JC, Baas DC, Beisekeeva J, et al. The dynamic nature of Bruch's membrane. Prog Retin Eye Res. 2010;29:1–18.

Borooah S, Phillips MJ, Bilican B, et al. Using human induced pluripotent stem cells to treat retinal disease. Prog Retin Eye Res. 2013;37:163–81.

Boyden ES, Zhang F, Bamberg E, et al. Millisecond-timescale, genetically targeted optical control of neural activity. Nat Neurosci. 2005;8:1263–8.

Buchholz DEH, Hikita ST, Rowland TJ, Friedrich AM, Hinman CR, Johnson LV, Clegg DO. Derivation of functional retinal pigmented epithelium from induced pluripotent stem cells. Stem Cells. 2009;10:2427–34.

Busskamp V, Duebel J, Balya D, et al. Genetic reactivation of cone photoreceptors restores visual responses in retinitis pigmentosa. Science. 2010;329:413–7.

Carr AJ, Vugler AA, Hikita ST, et al. Protective effects of human iPS-derived retinal pigment epithelium cell transplantation in the retinal dystrophic rat. PLoS One. 2009;4:e8152.

Cehajic-Kapetanovic J, Eleftheriou C, Allen AE, et al. Restoration of vision with ectopic expression of human rod opsin. Curr Biol. 2015;25:2111–22.

Chow BY, Han X, Dobry AS, et al. High-performance genetically targetable optical neural silencing by light-driven proton pumps. Nature. 2010;463:98–102.

Cideciyan AV, Hauswirth WW, Aleman TS, et al. Human RPE65 gene therapy for Leber congenital amaurosis: persistence of early visual improvements and safety at 1 year. Hum Gene Ther. 2009;20:999–1004.

Cosentino C, Alberio L, Gazzarrini S, et al. Optogenetics. Engineering of a light-gated potassium channel. Science. 2015;348:707–10.

Cronin T, Vandenberghe LH, Hantz P, et al. Efficient transduction and optogenetic stimulation of retinal bipolar cells by a synthetic adeno-associated virus capsid and promoter. EMBO Mol Med. 2014;6:1175–90.

Dalkara D, Byrne LC, Klimczak RR, et al. In vivo-directed evolution of a new adeno-associated virus for therapeutic outer retinal gene delivery from the vitreous. Sci Transl Med. 2013;5:189ra76.

Dalkara D, Goureau O, Marazova K, et al. Let there be light: gene and cell therapy for blindness. Hum Gene Ther. 2016;27:134–47.

Decembrini S, Koch U, Radtke F, et al. Derivation of traceable and transplantable photoreceptors from mouse embryonic stem cells. Stem Cell Rep. 2014;2:853–65.

Diniz KT, Cabral-Filho JE, Miranda RM, et al. Effect of the kangaroo position on the electromyographic activity of preterm children: a follow-up study. BMC Pediatr. 2013;13:79.

Doroudchi MM, Greenberg KP, Liu J, et al. Virally delivered channelrhodopsin-2 safely and effectively restores visual function in multiple mouse models of blindness. Mol Ther. 2011;19:1220–9.

Eiraku M, Takata N, Ishibashi H, et al. Self-organizing optic-cup morphogenesis in three-dimensional culture. Nature. 2011;472:51–6.

Forrester JV. Privilege revisited: an evaluation of the eye's defence mechanisms. Eye (Lond). 2009;23:756–66.

Fradot M, Busskamp V, Forster V, et al. Gene therapy in ophthalmology: validation on cultured retinal cells and explants from postmortem human eyes. Hum Gene Ther. 2011;22:587–93.

Garber K. RIKEN suspends first clinical trial involving induced pluripotent stem cells. Nat Biotechnol. 2015;33:890–1.

Garita-Hernandez M, Diaz-Corrales F, Lukovic D, et al. Hypoxia increases the yield of photoreceptors differentiating from mouse embryonic stem cells and improves the modeling of retinogenesis in vitro. Stem Cells. 2013;31:966–78.

Gaub BM, Berry MH, Holt AE, et al. Optogenetic vision restoration using rhodopsin for enhanced sensitivity. Mol Ther. 2015;23:1562–71.

Gonzalez-Cordero A, West EL, Pearson RA, et al. Photoreceptor precursors derived from three-dimensional embryonic stem cell cultures integrate and mature within adult degenerate retina. Nat Biotechnol. 2013;31:741–7.

Gouras P, Flood MT, Kjeldbye H. Transplantation of cultured human retinal cells to monkey retina. An Acad Bras Cienc. 1984;56:431–43.

Gouras P, Flood MT, Kjedbye H, et al. Transplantation of cultured human retinal epithelium to Bruch's membrane of the owl monkey's eye. Curr Eye Res. 1985;4:253–65.

Gourraud PA, Gilson L, Girard M, et al. The role of human leukocyte antigen matching in the development of multiethnic "haplobank" of induced pluripotent stem cell lines. Stem Cells. 2012;30:180–6.

Greenberg KP, Pham A, Werblin FS. Differential targeting of optical neuromodulators to ganglion cell soma and dendrites allows dynamic control of center-surround antagonism. Neuron. 2011;69:713–20.

Ham WT Jr, Ruffolo JJ Jr, Mueller HA, et al. Histologic analysis of photochemical lesions produced in rhesus retina by short-wave-length light. Invest Ophthalmol Vis Sci. 1978;17:1029–35.

Hausser M. Optogenetics: the age of light. Nat Methods. 2014;11:1012–4.

He H, Tan Y, Duffort S, et al. In vivo downregulation of innate and adaptive immune responses in corneal allograft rejection by HC-HA/PTX3 complex purified from amniotic membrane. Invest Ophthalmol Vis Sci. 2014;55:1647–56.

Hu Y, Liu L, Lu B, et al. A novel approach for subretinal implantation of ultrathin substrates containing stem cell-derived retinal pigment epithelium monolayer. Ophthalmic Res. 2012;48:186–91.

Ivanova E, Pan ZH. Evaluation of the adeno-associated virus mediated long-term expression of channelrhodopsin-2 in the mouse retina. Mol Vis. 2009;15:1680–9.

Ivanova E, Hwang GS, Pan ZH, et al. Evaluation of AAV-mediated expression of Chop2-GFP in the marmoset retina. Invest Ophthalmol Vis Sci. 2010;51:5288–96.

Jacobson SG, Cideciyan AV. Treatment possibilities for retinitis pigmentosa. N Engl J Med. 2010;363:1669–71.

Jha BS, Bharti K. Regenerating retinal pigment epithelial cells to cure blindness: a road towards personalized artificial tissue. Curr Stem Cell Rep. 2015;1:79–91.

Jones BW, Pfeiffer RL, Ferrell WD, et al. Retinal remodeling in human retinitis pigmentosa. Exp Eye Res. 2016;150:149–65.

Kador KE, Goldberg JL. Scaffolds and stem cells: delivery of cell transplants for retinal degenerations. Expert Rev Ophthalmol. 2012;7:459–70.

Kamao H, Mandai M, Okamoto S, et al. Characterization of human induced pluripotent stem cell-derived retinal pigment epithelium cell sheets aiming for clinical application. Stem Cell Rep. 2014;2:205–18.

Klapoetke NC, Murata Y, Kim SS, et al. Independent optical excitation of distinct neural populations. Nat Methods. 2014;11:338–46.

Klassen H. Stem cells in clinical trials for treatment of retinal degeneration. Expert Opin Biol Ther. 2016;16:7–14.

Kleinlogel S, Feldbauer K, Dempski RE, et al. Ultra light-sensitive and fast neuronal activation with the Ca(2)+-permeable channelrhodopsin CatCh. Nat Neurosci. 2011;14:513–8.

Krishnamoorthy V, Cherukuri P, Poria D, et al. Retinal remodeling: concerns, emerging remedies and future prospects. Front Cell Neurosci. 2016;10:38.

Kuwahara A, Ozone C, Nakano T, et al. Generation of a ciliary margin-like stem cell niche from self-organizing human retinal tissue. Nat Commun. 2015;6:6286.

Lagali PS, Balya D, Awatramani GB, et al. Light-activated channels targeted to ON bipolar cells restore visual function in retinal degeneration. Nat Neurosci. 2008;11:667–75.

Lamba DA, Gust J, Reh TA. Transplantation of human embryonic stem cell-derived photoreceptors restores some visual function in Crx-deficient mice. Cell Stem Cell. 2009;4:73–9.

Lamba DA, McUsic A, Hirata RK, et al. Generation, purification and transplantation of photoreceptors derived from human induced pluripotent stem cells. PLoS One. 2010;5:e8763.

Leach LL, Clegg DO. Concise review: making stem cells retinal: methods for deriving retinal pigment epithelium and implications for patients with ocular disease. Stem Cells. 2015;33:2363–73.

Lin B, Koizumi A, Tanaka N, et al. Restoration of visual function in retinal degeneration mice by ectopic expression of melanopsin. Proc Natl Acad Sci U S A. 2008;105:16009–14.

Lin JY, Knutsen PM, Muller A, et al. ReaChR: a red-shifted variant of channelrhodopsin enables deep transcranial optogenetic excitation. Nat Neurosci. 2013;16:1499–508.

Liu Z, Yu N, Holz FG, et al. Enhancement of retinal pigment epithelial culture characteristics and subretinal space tolerance of scaffolds with 200 nm fiber topography. Biomaterials. 2014;35:2837–50.

Lopez R, Gouras P, Kjeldbye H, et al. Transplanted retinal pigment epithelium modifies the retinal degeneration in the RCS rat. Invest Ophthalmol Vis Sci. 1989;30:586–8.

Lu B, Morgans CW, Girman S, et al. Neural stem cells derived by small molecules preserve vision. Transl Vis Sci Technol. 2013;2:1.

Lu B, Tai YC, Humayun MS. Microdevice-based cell therapy for age-related macular degeneration. Dev Ophthalmol. 2014;53:155–66.

Mace E, Caplette R, Marre O, et al. Targeting channelrhodopsin-2 to ON-bipolar cells with vitreally administered AAV restores ON and OFF visual responses in blind mice. Mol Ther. 2015;23:7–16.

MacLaren RE, Groppe M, Barnard AR, et al. Retinal gene therapy in patients with choroideremia: initial findings from a phase 1/2 clinical trial. Lancet. 2014;383:1129–37.

Maguire AM, Simonelli F, Pierce EA, et al. Safety and efficacy of gene transfer for Leber's congenital amaurosis. N Engl J Med. 2008;358:2240–8.

Marc R, Pfeiffer R, Jones B. Retinal prosthetics, optogenetics, and chemical photoswitches. ACS Chem Neurosci. 2014;5:895–901.

Maruotti J, Sripathi SR, Bharti K, et al. Small-molecule-directed, efficient generation of retinal pigment epithelium from human pluripotent stem cells. Proc Natl Acad Sci U S A. 2015;112:10950–5.

Matsuno-Yagi A, Mukohata Y. Two possible roles of bacteriorhodopsin; a comparative study of strains of Halobacterium halobium differing in pigmentation. Biochem Biophys Res Commun. 1977;78:237–43.

Meyer JS, Howden SE, Wallace KA, et al. Optic vesicle-like structures derived from human pluripotent stem cells facilitate a customized approach to retinal disease treatment. Stem Cells. 2011;29:1206–18.

Nagel G, Ollig D, Fuhrmann M, et al. Channelrhodopsin-1: a light-gated proton channel in green algae. Science. 2002;296:2395–8.

Nagel G, Szellas T, Huhn W, et al. Channelrhodopsin-2, a directly light-gated cation-selective membrane channel. Proc Natl Acad Sci U S A. 2003;100:13940–5.

Nakano T, Ando S, Takata N, et al. Self-formation of optic cups and storable stratified neural retina from human ESCs. Cell Stem Cell. 2012;10:771–85.

Nazari H, Zhang L, Zhu D, et al. Stem cell based therapies for age-related macular degeneration: the promises and the challenges. Prog Retin Eye Res. 2015;48:1–39.

Niknejad H, Peirovi H, Jorjani M, et al. Properties of the amniotic membrane for potential use in tissue engineering. Eur Cell Mater. 2008;15:88–99.

Oesterhelt D, Stoeckenius W. Rhodopsin-like protein from the purple membrane of Halobacterium halobium. Nat New Biol. 1971;233:149–52.

Organisciak DT, Vaughan DK. Retinal light damage: mechanisms and protection. Prog Retin Eye Res. 2010;29:113–34.

Pan ZH, Ganjawala TH, Lu Q, et al. ChR2 mutants at L132 and T159 with improved operational light sensitivity for vision restoration. PLoS One. 2014;9:e98924.

Phillips MJ, Wallace KA, Dickerson SJ, et al. Blood-derived human iPS cells generate optic vesicle-like structures with the capacity to form retinal laminae and develop synapses. Invest Ophthalmol Vis Sci. 2012;53:2007–19.

Polosukhina A, Litt J, Tochitsky I, et al. Photochemical restoration of visual responses in blind mice. Neuron. 2012;75:271–82.

Ramsden CM, Powner MB, Carr AJ, et al. Stem cells in retinal regeneration: past, present and future. Development. 2013;140:2576–85.

Reh TA, Lamba D, Gust J. Directing human embryonic stem cells to a retinal fate. Methods Mol Biol. 2010;636:139–53.

Reichman S, Terray A, Slembrouck A, et al. From confluent human iPS cells to self-forming neural retina and retinal pigmented epithelium. Proc Natl Acad Sci U S A. 2014;111(23):8518.

Rozanowska M, Jarvis-Evans J, Korytowski W, et al. Blue light-induced reactivity of retinal age pigment. In vitro generation of oxygen-reactive species. J Biol Chem. 1995;270:18825–30.

Salero E, Blenkinsop TA, Corneo B, et al. Adult human RPE can be activated into a multipotent stem cell that produces mesenchymal derivatives. Cell Stem Cell. 2012;10:88–95.

Schwartz SD, Hubschman JP, Heilwell G, et al. Embryonic stem cell trials for macular degeneration: a preliminary report. Lancet. 2012;379:713–20.

Schwartz SD, Regillo CD, Lam BL, et al. Human embryonic stem cell-derived retinal pigment epithelium in patients with age-related macular degeneration and Stargardt's macular dystrophy: follow-up of two open-label phase 1/2 studies. Lancet. 2015;385:509–16.

Shirai H, Mandai M, Matsushita K, et al. Transplantation of human embryonic stem cell-derived retinal tissue in two primate models of retinal degeneration. Proc Natl Acad Sci U S A. 2016;113:E81–90.

Simonelli F, Maguire AM, Testa F, et al. Gene therapy for Leber's congenital amaurosis is safe and effective through 1.5 years after vector administration. Mol Ther. 2010;18:643–50.

Song MJ, Bharti K. Looking into the future: using induced pluripotent stem cells to build two and three dimensional ocular tissue for cell therapy and disease modeling. Brain Res. 2016;1638:2–14.

Song WK, Park KM, Kim HJ, et al. Treatment of macular degeneration using embryonic stem cell-derived retinal pigment epithelium: preliminary results in Asian patients. Stem Cell Rep. 2015;4:860–72.

Stanzel BV, Liu Z, Somboonthanakij S, et al. Human RPE stem cells grown into polarized RPE monolayers on a polyester matrix are maintained after grafting into rabbit subretinal space. Stem Cell Rep. 2014;2:64–77.

Strauss O. The retinal pigment epithelium in visual function. Physiol Rev. 2005;85:845–81.

Streilein JW, Ma N, Wenkel H, et al. Immunobiology and privilege of neuronal retina and pigment epithelium transplants. Vis Res. 2002;42:487–95.

Takahashi K, Tanabe K, Ohnuki M, et al. Induction of pluripotent stem cells from adult human fibroblasts by defined factors. Cell. 2007;131:861–72.

Taylor CJ, Bolton EM, Pocock S, et al. Banking on human embryonic stem cells: estimating the number of donor cell lines needed for HLA matching. Lancet. 2005;366:2019–25.

Thomson JA, Itskovitz-Eldor J, Shapiro SS, et al. Embryonic stem cell lines derived from human blastocysts. Science. 1998;282:1145–7.

Tochitsky I, Polosukhina A, Degtyar VE, et al. Restoring visual function to blind mice with a photoswitch that exploits electrophysiological remodeling of retinal ganglion cells. Neuron. 2014;81:800–13.

Tomita H, Sugano E, Yawo H, et al. Restoration of visual response in aged dystrophic RCS rats using AAV-mediated channelopsin-2 gene transfer. Invest Ophthalmol Vis Sci. 2007;48:3821–6.

Tomita H, Sugano E, Fukazawa Y, et al. Visual properties of transgenic rats harboring the channelrhodopsin-2 gene regulated by the thy-1.2 promoter. PLoS One. 2009;4:e7679.

Tomita H, Sugano E, Isago H, et al. Channelrhodopsin-2 gene transduced into retinal ganglion cells restores functional vision in genetically blind rats. Exp Eye Res. 2010;90:429–36.

Tomkins-Netzer O, Taylor SR, Bar A, et al. Treatment with repeat dexamethasone implants results in long-term disease control in eyes with noninfectious uveitis. Ophthalmology. 2014;121:1649–54.

Tsai Y, Lu B, Bakondi B, et al. Human iPSC-derived neural progenitors preserve vision in an AMD-like model. Stem Cells. 2015;33:2537–49.

Tucker BA, Park IH, Qi SD, et al. Transplantation of adult mouse iPS cell-derived photoreceptor precursors restores retinal structure and function in degenerative mice. PLoS One. 2011;6:e18992.

Wang S, Lu B, Wood P, et al. Grafting of ARPE-19 and Schwann cells to the subretinal space in RCS rats. Invest Ophthalmol Vis Sci. 2005;46:2552–60.

Wang S, Girman S, Lu B, et al. Long-term vision rescue by human neural progenitors in a rat model of photoreceptor degeneration. Invest Ophthalmol Vis Sci. 2008;49:3201–6.

West EL, Gonzalez-Cordero A, Hippert C, et al. Defining the integration capacity of embryonic stem cell-derived photoreceptor precursors. Stem Cells. 2012;30:1424–35.

Wiley LA, Burnight ER, Songstad AE, et al. Patient-specific induced pluripotent stem cells (iPSCs) for the study and treatment of retinal degenerative diseases. Prog Retin Eye Res. 2015;44:15–35.

Wong WL, Su X, Li X, et al. Global prevalence of age-related macular degeneration and disease burden projection for 2020 and 2040: a systematic review and meta-analysis. Lancet Glob Health. 2014;2:e106–16.

Wu J, Seregard S, Algvere PV. Photochemical damage of the retina. Surv Ophthalmol. 2006;51:461–81.

van Wyk M, Pielecka-Fortuna J, Lowel S, et al. Restoring the ON switch in blind retinas: opto-mGluR6, a next-generation, cell-tailored optogenetic tool. PLoS Biol. 2015;13:e1002143.

Zhang Y, Ivanova E, Bi A, et al. Ectopic expression of multiple microbial rhodopsins restores ON and OFF light responses in retinas with photoreceptor degeneration. J Neurosci. 2009;29:9186–96.

Zhong X, Gutierrez C, Xue T, et al. Generation of three-dimensional retinal tissue with functional photoreceptors from human iPSCs. Nat Commun. 2014;5:4047.

Zhou L, Wang W, Liu Y, et al. Differentiation of induced pluripotent stem cells of swine into rod photoreceptors and their integration into the retina. Stem Cells. 2011;29:972–80.

Index

© Springer International Publishing AG 2018
M.S. Humayun, L.C. Olmos de Koo (eds.), *Retinal Prosthesis*, Essentials in
Ophthalmology, https://doi.org/10.1007/978-3-319-67260-1

The manufacturer's authorised representative in the EU is Springer
Nature Customer Service Centre GmbH, Europaplatz 3, 69115 Heidelberg,
Germany. If you have any concerns regarding our products, please
contact ProductSafety@springernature.com

Printed and bound by CPI Group (UK) Ltd, Croydon, CR0 4YY

23/04/2026

02095596-0004